Is Marijuana The Right Medicine For You?

Is Marijuana The Right Medicine For You?

A FACTUAL GUIDE TO THE MEDICAL USES OF MARIJUANA

Bill Zimmerman, PhD
with Rick Bayer, MD
and Nancy Crumpacker, MD

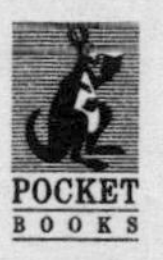

LONDON · SYDNEY · NEW YORK · TOKYO · SINGAPORE · TORONTO

First published in the USA by Keats Publishing Inc, 1998
First published in Great Britain by Pocket Books, 1999
An imprint of Simon & Schuster UK Ltd
A Viacom Company

1 3 5 7 9 10 8 6 4 2

Simon & Schuster UK Ltd
Africa House
64–78 Kingsway
London WC2B 6AH

Simon & Schuster Australia
Sydney

A CIP catalogue record for this book is available from the British Library

ISBN 0-671-03396-4

Typeset in Goudy by SX Composing DTP, Rayleigh, Essex
Printed and bound in Great Britain by
Caledonian International Book Manufacturing Ltd, Glasgow

Contents

Acknowledgements

Gina Pesulima and Dave Fratello played an invaluable role in the preparation of this book. Ms Pesulima, a superb writer, coordinated the research, interviewing and editing. Mr Fratello, who served as Communications Director during the Proposition 215 campaign in California, and serves today in the same capacity for Americans for Medical Rights, contributed his expertise, historical knowledge and communications skills. Both deserve much of the credit for the quality of the final product.

Preface

Don't read this entire book. It isn't necessary. Since it is written for patients, their caregivers and their loved ones, the book is organized to allow readers to cut to the chase, to quickly find information relevant to a particular disease category or set of symptoms. We assume that if you are reading this book to find out how to use marijuana to relieve the symptoms of glaucoma, you may not be particularly interested in how it alleviates the side-effects of cancer chemotherapy.

The best way to read this book is to start with the introduction and the first three chapters. This will give you important background information you will need later. Then look in the table of contents and find the chapter that covers the particular disease or set of symptoms that affects you or your loved one. Read that chapter next. Then read the last five chapters of the book. These chapters will give you information you will need to know before actually obtaining and using marijuana.

Introduction

Few topics generate as much controversy as marijuana. Millions of people believe it is a dangerous drug capable of undermining the social order. Millions of others believe it is relatively benign, and far less harmful than legal drugs like alcohol and nicotine. People in the first category support current laws that make the possession or use of marijuana a crime punishable by fines and imprisonment. Many in the second category think such laws do more harm than good, and that society would be better off if marijuana were legal.

Both sides in this debate often exaggerate the facts used to support their arguments. The debate is about the nonmedical or recreational use of marijuana, but it has had an enormous impact on discussions of medical use. In this brief introduction we will present some of the arguments about recreational use and some of the facts you may find helpful in making up your own mind about marijuana.

To be fair, we first need to disclose our own backgrounds and biases. Bill Zimmerman was trained as a scientist in the area of neuropsychology, and received a PhD from the University of Chicago in 1967. Later he served on the faculties of the University of Chicago and Brooklyn College in New York. He is now a partner in the political consulting firm, Zimmerman and Markman, based in Santa Monica, California. He managed the successful 1996 Proposition 215 campaign in California, the first time a state voted to authorize the medical use of marijuana. He is currently the director of Americans for Medical Rights, an organization working to place similar voter initiatives on ballots across the country.

Rick Bayer earned his medical degree from the University of Missouri at Kansas City in 1978. He performed his postgraduate training at Oregon Health Sciences University in Portland, Oregon, and is board certified by the American Board of Internal Medicine. He was in the private practice of primary care internal medicine for fifteen years before incurring a medical disability. He then became active in Oregon politics and is currently assisting a campaign in Oregon to help pass legislation that would permit medical patients to use marijuana. He is a member of the American Medical Association, the American Public Health Association, the American College of Physicians, and Physicians for Social Responsibility.

Nancy Crumpacker received her medical degree from the University of Kansas in 1975. She did her postgraduate training in internal medicine at Truman Medical Center in Kansas City and her medical oncology fellowship at Oregon Health Sciences University in Portland. She is board certified in internal medicine and medical oncology and primarily treats people with cancer. She is a member of the American Society of Clinical Oncology, American College of Physicians, and Physicians for Social Responsibility. Nancy Crumpacker and Rick Bayer are married and live together in Portland.

All of us firmly believe that marijuana has legitimate medical uses. Later in this book, we will present ample evidence to support that belief. But meanwhile many readers may not have had prior personal experience using marijuana, either for medical or recreational purposes, and may be justifiably reluctant or even afraid to consider using it as a medicine. We feel it is important to address these fears and shed some light on this very polarized debate before discussing the medicinal use of marijuana.

Those who support criminal sanctions against the use of marijuana believe the plant has many dangerous qualities. For example, they often claim that even though marijuana is considered a 'soft' drug, it is nonetheless addictive, in much the same way that 'hard' drugs like heroin and cocaine are addictive. Those who favour legalizing marijuana point out that 70 million Americans have tried it. In the UK, it is estimated that 6 million people have used cannabis at some time, while 1.25 to 2.75 million are thought to smoke it regularly. If it were truly addictive, tens of millions would still be hooked, a statement that clearly cannot be supported.

Many who favour legalization will readily admit that for a minority of marijuana users, there may be some physiological or psychological dependence. Nevertheless, this has to be taken in context. Caffeine, nicotine, alcohol, marijuana, cocaine and heroin are six addictive drugs in common use throughout the Western world. Some are legal, some are not. When physicians and scientists are asked to compare these six drugs in terms of how addictive each is relative to the others, there is a surprising consensus. Heroin is commonly believed to be the most addictive substance, but many doctors believe that alcohol and nicotine are as addictive as heroin or very close to it. Cocaine generally comes next, followed by caffeine. Virtually all of them believe marijuana to be the least addictive of the six (Mathre, 1997; 180).

Supporters of criminal sanctions against marijuana also claim that it is a 'gateway' drug. That means that while marijuana itself may be only slightly harmful, using it sometimes leads to involvement with harder drugs. However, marijuana legalizers point out that ever since the 1950s, there have been a fairly consistent 500,000 heroin addicts in the US. Marijuana use was minimal in that decade but virtually exploded in the next. If marijuana leads to heroine, they ask, why wasn't there a massive increase in heroin addicts following the massive increase in marijuana users? Similarly, there have been roughly 160,000 heroin addicts in the UK for the last 5 to 10 years. While numbers of marijuana smokers have jumped significantly (by about 1 million in 5 years), the number of hard drug addicts has remained steady.

The antimarijuana forces believe that while casual marijuana use may not lead to negative health effects, prolonged use disrupts psychological functioning and physical health. Various claims have been made that such prolonged use harms the immune system, causes cancer, disrupts reproductive function, leads to mental illness and a host of other adverse outcomes. There is no scientific evidence to support these claims.

Scientists have studied working-class men in Jamaica who smoke ganja (the local name for marijuana) in large quantities every day of their lives. Some smoked as many as a dozen marijuana cigarettes every day for decades. Extensive batteries of physiological and psychological tests performed on these individuals revealed no differences from the population at large (Comitas, 1976).

There is one area, however, where the pro- and anti-marijuana forces agree. Children should not use marijuana recreationally. There is also agreement that inhaling any type of smoke can cause respiratory problems. Of course, many medical patients have more pressing concerns than the possible side-effects that may result from inhaling a few puffs of smoke each day.

We are not endorsing the use of marijuana for recreational purposes. Rather, we want to place claims about the dangers of marijuana in a context helpful to medical patients contemplating its use. One way to do that is to consider the possibility of a lethal overdose. There are records of marijuana use that literally go back thousands of years. It was used by ancient civilizations across the globe, and is in common use on every continent today. Yet, there has never been a lethal overdose due to marijuana.

Many drugs are lethal when taken in excessive quantity. It is common knowledge that one can die from taking too many tranquillizers or sleeping pills. Moreover, everyone has heard of hard drug users dying from an overdose of heroin. It is less commonly known that a person can die from taking excessive amounts of aspirin or paracetamol (Hedex, Panadol, Disprin, Calpol, etc.), but it is true. Yet, there is no amount of marijuana that is lethal, regardless of the quantity consumed. As every marijuana user knows, if you smoke or eat too much, you simply fall asleep. However, there are isolated reports of new marijuana users experiencing anxiety or panic attacks because of their lack of familiarity with the psychological effects of the drug. We will discuss this problem in greater detail in a later chapter.

Marijuana was first made illegal in the United States in 1937. As far back as the Civil War, doctors commonly prescribed it for pain relief and other ailments. Its use declined around the turn of the century when more powerful drugs, like morphine and other opiates (drugs derived from the opium poppy plant), became available. Later, in the early 1970s, the US government further defined its antidrug policies with the passage of the Controlled Substances Act that is still in force today.

The Controlled Substances Act governs US law with respect to drug use and controls which drugs doctors can and cannot prescribe. It defines five categories of drugs, called Schedules. Schedule I drugs are deemed to be dangerous, and to have no legitimate medical use. As a result, doctors are not permitted to prescribe them and pharmacies are not permitted to stock them. Schedule II drugs are also deemed to be dangerous, but are recognized as having some legitimate medical use. Doctors are permitted to prescribe Schedule II drugs but must observe very tight controls and procedures in doing so. Drugs in Schedules III, IV and V are successively less dangerous and doctors have greater flexibility in prescribing or recommending them.

Marijuana was placed in Schedule I, along with heroin and LSD. Morphine, cocaine and methamphetamine are in Schedule II. Advocates for the medical use of marijuana believe that marijuana is far less dangerous than Schedule II drugs like morphine, cocaine and methamphetamine. Further, we believe that marijuana does, in fact, have many legitimate medical uses. Therefore, we think that the government should remove marijuana from Schedule I and place it in Schedule II. Such a move would instantly allow doctors to prescribe marijuana for appropriate patients, and allow patients to legally obtain it in pharmacies. If this rescheduling took place at the federal level, there would no longer be a need for state laws, like ballot initiatives, to address the problem.

In 1974, a citizens group filed a suit demanding that marijuana be moved to Schedule II. The US government was able to block any action on this suit for over a decade. Finally, in 1986, hearings began before administrative law judge Francis L. Young of the Drug Enforcement Administration (DEA) to determine the facts surrounding the medical use of marijuana. Those hearings went on for two years. At their conclusion, Judge Young ruled in favour of moving marijuana to Schedule II. He said that marijuana met the standards of 'currently accepted medical use in treatment in the United States'. He also stated, on the record, that 'marijuana, in its natural form, is one of the safest therapeutically active substances known to man.'

Following Judge Young's decision, the Administrator of the

DEA overruled him. For political, rather than medical, reasons, marijuana has remained in Schedule I ever since.

Cannabis has been illegal in the UK since the 1925 Geneva International Convention on Narcotics Control. Until 1971, however, it was legitimately prescribed for medicinal purposes. The 1971 Misuse of Drugs Act, which is still in force today, makes it illegal for doctors to prescribe this drug, and for people to possess, grow or take it. Regulations made under the Act of 1971 enable the Home Secretary to issue licences for the cultivation of cannabis plants and even for the smoking of it, but only 'for the purpose of research'.

In the UK, government regulations determine the degree of availability of many substances that have an abuse potential. Regulated drugs are also classified by how harmful they are when abused. The Misuse of Drugs Act 1971 prohibits activities relating to the manufacture, sale and possession of particular drugs. The drugs are graded in three classes according to their harmfulness if misused. Offences that involve Class A drugs, potentially the most harmful when abused, carry the highest penalties, while those involving Class C drugs carry the lowest penalties. Marijuana is currently classed in the B group. Cannabis and cannabis resin have the distinction of being the only ones on a short list of Class B controlled drugs for which there is no approved medicinal use and the prescribing of which is prohibited with no available exemption.

The Misuse of Drugs Regulations 1985 define those people who are authorized in their professional capacity to supply and possess controlled drugs. The Regulations also describe the requirements for legally undertaking these activities, such as storage of the drugs and limits on their prescription. Drugs are divided into five schedules based on their potential for abuse if misused.

In Schedule I, which includes marijuana, virtually all of the drugs are prohibited, except in accordance with Home Office authority. All of them have high potential for abuse and are not used medicinally.

We believe that the answer to the ongoing international debates in the UK and the US about the medical use of marijuana is to remove it from Schedule I and place it in Schedule II. This does not require the government or anyone else to take a position on legalizing marijuana for nonmedical use. In this book, we take no position on such recreational use. However, we do believe that if marijuana can alleviate disease, the symptoms of disease, or side-effects of prescription drugs, it can be tried without undue anxiety about harmful side-effects.

We conclude this introduction with a quote from a commentary written by Harvard professor Lester Grinspoon, which was published in the *Journal of the American Medical Association* on 21 June 1995:

> One of marijuana's greatest advantages as a medicine is its remarkable safety. It has little effect on major physiological functions. There is no known case of a lethal overdose . . . Marijuana is also far less addictive and far less subject to abuse than many drugs now used as muscle relaxants, hypnotics, and analgesics . . . The ostensible indifference of physicians should no longer be used as a justification for keeping this medicine in the shadows.

Since this book has the narrow purpose of assisting medical patients, we will not again discuss the recreational side of marijuana. For readers who want more information on this subject, we recommend *Marijuana Myths, Marijuana Facts* by Lynn Zimmer, PhD and John Morgan, MD. It is currently the most scientifically reliable book available on the psychological and health implications of long term marijuana use.

Chapter 1
Herbal Medicine: Folk Remedies to Modern Science

In February 1997, the National Institutes of Health, a federally funded agency in the US, hosted a conference on the medical uses of marijuana. It was shortly after the passage of Proposition 215, the medical marijuana law, in California. During a public comment portion of the session, a doctor from Arizona, who described himself as an addiction psychiatrist, argued against government approval for any new research on medical marijuana. He believed it would be a step backwards for science to undertake research on a crude plant. He said that if such research led to government approval for marijuana, it would be unique in the modern pharmacopoeia (the totality of drugs approved for therapeutic use). He pointed out, with obvious satisfaction, that modern science had supplanted all crude plant remedies with pure chemical compounds.

In the audience, a breast cancer survivor from California listened sceptically. She had come to the conference to explain how marijuana had helped her get through the wrenching nausea caused by her chemotherapy. In response to the addiction psychiatrist, she rose to make a different point. She said that for some women, bladder infections were a common problem. In the past, she continued, these infections would be treated with prescription drugs. Nowadays, she said, most women she knew drank cranberry juice instead, because it usually works better and has fewer or no side-effects.

This little episode illustrates one of the central problems in the debate about the medical use of marijuana. Ancient and traditional medicine, lacking the ability to isolate and manufacture pure chemicals, was based primarily on natural remedies provided by plants. As late as the first decades of this century, doctors often relied on the accumulated wisdom of the ages when they recommended various plants or plant extracts to cure disease and alleviate symptoms. Modern medicine operates very differently.

As a result of discoveries made in the last hundred years, doctors today are armed with a dazzling array of chemical weapons in their war against disease. But each of these 'cures' or 'symptom relievers' consists of a single isolated chemical, usually a synthetic substance manufactured in a laboratory. Aside from the obvious and spectacular progress that has been made in the fight against disease, reliance on single isolated chemicals has other advantages.

Isolated chemicals can be scientifically tested. The scientific method requires that all factors capable of influencing a particular phenomenon be held constant in order to assess the impact of the single factor being tested. For example, to test the effectiveness of an experimental drug, two similar groups of patients are assembled. Their chemical intake is kept as identical as possible, except one group is given the drug to be tested and the other is given a 'placebo', a drug that looks, smells and tastes like the experimental drug but is, in fact, chemically inert. If differences show up between the two groups, they are attributed to the experimental drug. This is called a 'controlled' experiment because all factors but one, the experimental drug, are controlled by the researchers.

This method of testing the effects of drugs is very powerful. It allows researchers to say with relative certainty that a particular drug (isolated chemical compound) will have a specific effect on a particular set of patients at certain dosage levels. The scientific method is so powerful, in fact, that virtually all of modern Western medicine is based on it.

Cranberry juice, however, cannot be rigorously tested using the scientific method. Neither can marijuana. Both substances are made up of numerous chemical compounds. Smoked marijuana, for example, contains over 400 different, chemical compounds. One of those compounds is cellulose, the stiff, starchy material that gives plant stems their rigidity. Another is chlorophyll, the chemical that allows the plant to convert sunlight into energy needed for growth. A third is delta-9-tetrahydrocannabinol (THC), one of the chemicals in marijuana that binds to brain sites and produces many of the psychological effects of the drug. Scientists studying the medicinal properties of marijuana – or cranberry juice – would be unable to tell which of these many compounds was producing the desired effect.

This inability causes other problems, having to do with the manufacture and sale of medicines, which further explains why our medical system is dependent upon single isolated chemical compounds. In America, the Federal Food and Drug Administration (FDA) was established to test the safety and usefulness of substances consumed by humans. To begin research on a new drug, with the intent of gaining FDA approval for sale and distribution, a pharmaceutical company must initiate a 'New Drug Application'. If controlled scientific research, paid for by the company, shows the drug to be safe and effective, the company receives a patent on the substance and a monopoly on its production and sale for a number of years.

It takes many years to complete a New Drug Application and bring a drug to the market for sale. The research and development often costs over a hundred million dollars to complete. In the UK, the supply and use of medicines is based on the Medicines Act 1968. This means that any product for which a medicinal claim is made must be licensed by the government. The Committee on Safety of Medicines, whose members include independent experts, advises ministers on the licensing of medicines. The whole system is administered by the Medicines Control Agency, a branch of the Department of Health.

The Medicines Control Agency is responsible for seeing that all medicines supplied or sold for human or animal use in Britain meet certain standards. Before a medicine is marketed, as much information must be known about its quality, effectiveness and safety as possible. Laboratory and animal studies provide information on the drugs effectiveness, as well as its possible harmful effects. Then the drug must be studied in 2000–3000 people, both those who need treatment and healthy volunteers. When the tests and trials are finished, the pharmaceutical company can apply to the Medicines Control Agency for a licence. The information about the medicine that has been recorded over the years of its development is sent to the Medicines Control Agency for assessment.

The EU is moving steadily towards a single market in pharmaceuticals. Proposals on drug licensing, distribution, pricing, labelling and patient information have all been considered, and some have been implemented.

The Medicines Control Agency has been working with other European drug regulatory bodies towards the single internal market. Three systems for licensing medicines are now available to the pharmaceutical industry: a centralized system, a decentralized system and a single application system. A single centralized European medicines agency, the European Medicines Evaluation Agency (EMEA) based in London, deals with applications for new chemical entities and products of biotechnology. A committee of scientific experts (Committee of Proprietary Medicinal Products – CPMP) is responsible for assessing each application for a product licence. The EMEA gives the final approval for a licence based on the recommendations of the CPMP. A licence granted by this route is then valid in all member states of the European Union. The EMEA will monitor drug safety after the medicine is marketed.

The new centralized system may bring greater openness with the publication of an assessment report outlining the reasons for licensing a product. The Medicines Act, on which the licensing of medicines is based in the UK, makes it a criminal offence for MCA officials to reveal any information having to do with a licence application. An attempt to amend this section of the Medicines Act through a private member's bill in 1993 failed. Finding out why medicines are licensed or withdrawn for use in Britain remains impossible, in stark contrast to the US, where the FDA allows this sort of disclosure to the public.

Whatever the route that a pharmaceutical company takes to license a product, an enormous amount of money and time is spent. In 1988, the average size of a dossier of information on one drug was 170 volumes, each the dimension of a telephone directory. Development of a new drug may take 10 years, and cost the pharmaceutical company in the region of £150 million. Every year over £3.5 billion of pharmaceuticals are consumed. How much money pharmaceutical companies make from selling medicines has always been a secret between them and the Department of Health, but there is no question that pharmaceuticals and, in particular, a successful drug, are big, big business.

A drug company can only invest that kind of time and money if there is an opportunity to earn enough profit to recoup its investment. Generally, such profits can only be made if the company has the exclusive right to market the drug, that is, if it has a patent on its manufacture. Also, to protect it from lawsuits that could sap profits, the company must be able to show that it did responsible scientific research proving the claims it subsequently made on behalf of the new drug.

You can see the problem. Plants are not drugs as the term is commonly understood in our system of medicine. Plants are never made up of single chemical compounds. Plants cannot be manufactured. A drug company cannot take out a patent on a plant. Mother Nature already has one. Therefore, a drug company cannot hope for a marketing monopoly on a plant. As a result, the sale and distribution of medicinal plants does not present drug companies with the same financial opportunities they have with single isolated chemicals.

Of course, it is possible to do research on the medicinal properties of plants. However, that research will rarely be as scientifically rigorous as research done on single isolated chemicals. For example, a scientist could test the effectiveness of cranberry juice in curing bladder infections. The researcher would isolate two groups of women with bladder infections and for several days feed them the same diets and keep them in the same living conditions. One group would get cranberry juice and the other group a different kind of juice. After several days, the researcher would ask each group to report their symptoms and indicate whether or not those symptoms had decreased, increased or stayed constant.

The results of such an experiment would be valid, but not conclusive. Some of the women in the experiment might already be aware that cranberry juice is supposed to treat bladder infections. Their taste buds would tell them whether or not they had received cranberry juice in the experiment, and that knowledge might colour what they said about their own symptoms when the experiment ended. The researchers conducting the study would question the validity of the results because the experimental subjects knew what product they were receiving. This study would only test the effectiveness of a common food. Since drug companies cannot obtain exclusive licensing patents on common foods, the drug companies would ignore the study.

Despite these many factors working against the use and distribution of natural plant remedies, there is currently an exploding public interest in such remedies and in ancient and Eastern healing practices. While many physicians frown on such remedies, many do not, and patients everywhere are discovering that in certain circumstances they do produce the desired benefit. That may seem like a sharp turn away from modern medicine, but keep in mind that these ancient practices were commonplace only two or three generations ago.

This renewed interest in natural remedies results from two factors. First is the widespread rediscovery that under certain circumstances some of these natural remedies actually work. Second is the growing realization that there are substantial risks in allowing synthetic substances of any kind into the body, whether they are drugs, food additives, pesticide residues or pollutants.

The rediscovery of natural remedies may seem less surprising if you consider that at least one out of every four synthetic drugs manufactured by drug companies today is ultimately derived from a plant. Many physicians and patients are simply starting to wonder why we don't go back to the plants themselves and re-examine their healing properties.

There are numerous examples of whole plant medicines returning to widespread use. The succulent aloe vera, a cactus-like plant, has been broadly accepted for nearly two decades as a skin application. It is used to help heal cuts and scrapes, as an antibacterial agent and as a topical moisturizer. Many households now grow a few of these plants in window pots.

When children or grown-ups need skin repair, they clip off a piece and apply the liquid inside to the affected area. Extracts of the plant are commonly used as additives in skin lotions and shampoos. Some believe that high concentrations of Vitamin E are the reason why aloe vera seems to work. However, like marijuana – and cranberry juice – there are hundreds of compounds in that liquid.

Echinacea is a natural herb taken by millions to prevent diseases like the common cold. The Chinese ginseng root is marketed widely to boost mental clarity and energy. Doctors and nutritionists encourage people to eat foods like carrots and sweet potatoes that contain beta-carotene (or carotin) as a way of protecting themselves against cancer. Broccoli is recommended for the same purpose. Garlic is now recognized for several beneficial effects, including reducing cholesterol. Why put a synthetic chemical in your body when you can sprinkle chopped garlic on your food instead?

The medicinal use of marijuana should be understood in this context. Unfortunately, the issue is clouded by the fact that in addition to effectively reducing many uncomfortable symptoms, marijuana also produces a psychological 'high'. Marijuana alters mood, and therefore must be considered an intoxicant. This makes many people more reluctant to use it than they otherwise might be. But does this perception have merit? Years ago doctors regularly told their patients that there might be health benefits if they drank a glass or two of wine every day, or had a daily shot of whisky. We now know that a daily glass of wine will decrease the risk of heart attacks. Such advice might have gone unheeded if it was marijuana being recommended, but what, in fact, is the difference?

Recently, another herb with mind-altering qualities has come into widespread use in the United States and Europe – precisely because of its affect on mood. St John's Wort, a herb of Scottish origin, is generating a great deal of excitement as an antidepressant. The plant, whose extract is known by the Latin term Hypericum, is already the biggest selling antidepressant in Germany, outselling the pharmaceutical, Prozac, by an estimated 20-to-1 margin. In the rest of the Western world, books are being written about it, web sites are devoted to it, and health food shops are selling it.

Patients taking St John's Wort for the required two- to six-week start-up regime report mood stabilization, and even general feelings of happiness while continuing to use the plant. Perhaps more importantly, many claim that they do not suffer any of the unpleasant side-effects that are sometimes associated with Prozac and the other synthetic chemicals now sold as antidepressants. Even scientists from the American FDA have become interested, and research into this herb in the UK has also begun. They recently announced the beginning of controlled clinical trials on St John's Wort. Too bad marijuana can't get the same treatment.

With traditional plant medicines like St John's Wort undergoing testing as treatments for distinctly modern ailments like depression, marijuana places the modern scientific testing process in a curious position. It is hard to argue that the drug authorities should not be as open to the benefits of marijuana as it is to those of St John's Wort. After all, marijuana is believed by many to alleviate symptoms and conditions every bit as serious as depression.

Unfortunately, the difference is neither scientific nor medical. It is political. Thousands of patients across America, the UK and Europe are hoping that in the coming years their governments will be able to take the politics out of the medical marijuana issue and deal with it solely as a scientific issue.

In the meantime, readers thinking about the medicinal use of marijuana should not only put the politics aside, but also leave behind any prejudicial attitudes they may still have about herbal medicine and natural remedies. Isolated synthetic chemicals are not the only way to effectively treat disease and alleviate symptoms.

As Dr James Gordon, Professor of Psychiatry and Family Medicine at Georgetown University, Washington, DC, said on 10 October 1997 to the US Senate Subcommittee on Public Health and Safety:

> For tens of millions of Americans, it is no longer a question of either modern science or ancient wisdom, but of combining both in a new, richer, more effective and more humane synthesis.

Chapter 2
Marijuana: Not a Cure, But a Way to Reduce Symptoms

Marijuana is not a miracle drug. It does not 'cure' disease. However, for some patients, it can bring about near-miraculous relief from symptoms that other prescription or over-the-counter drugs are unable to alleviate.

Marijuana does not work for everyone. Some patients report achieving significant relief after using marijuana. Others, with exactly the same problem, claim that no relief is gained.

Even if it does work well, marijuana may not be the most effective source of relief for certain disorders or for certain people. It is one thing to say that a drug like marijuana reduces symptoms. It is another thing to claim that it is the most effective way to reduce those symptoms. We believe that patients should consider a wide variety of solutions for their individual problems. They should also watch for new developments. Some patients who have found that marijuana is the most effective medicine for them may discover later that something better has been put on the market.

We also believe that a patient's subjective judgement about the effectiveness of any medicine, including marijuana, must be taken seriously. Too many doctors are too quick to write off patient claims about the effectiveness of marijuana by saying, 'It's just their imagination.' No one can ever be certain whether such claims are imaginary or not. Keep in mind that one of the most important goals of medicine, if not the most important goal, is to relieve human suffering. When it comes to cures, doctors are often able to make objective measurements of success. However, when the goal is symptom control, only the patient is able to judge accurately the effectiveness of treatment.

Wherever possible, patients should use marijuana under medical supervision. The use of marijuana should always be considered a therapeutic trial just like any other prescription drug. Since marijuana works for some patients and not for others, it is impossible for the doctor or the patient to know in advance whether it will produce the desired effect. Each individual is unique and therefore each individual must conduct their own trial. Doctors should be willing to tolerate and even encourage such trials. If one's doctor refuses to conduct this therapeutic trial, the patient may question the doctor's commitment to relieve human suffering and may wish to seek another doctor. Never let social or political bias of your doctor interfere with your ability to find an effective medicine.

Marijuana is a very versatile drug. It is capable of helping patients with a very wide range of symptoms. It can be used to reduce adverse side-effects caused by other drugs. It can be used either alone or in combination with other medicines to reduce painful or undesirable symptoms. It can also be used to prevent the onset of such symptoms or side-effects. Finally, it can help the body function more normally when disease has disrupted various physiological functions.

In later chapters, we will describe in detail the most common uses of marijuana, especially in the treatment of severe medical conditions. We will focus on the ways marijuana has helped patients through difficult treatments for AIDS and cancer, how it has perhaps saved the sight of some glaucoma patients, and how regular doses of marijuana seem to have prevented patients from experiencing the most severe effects of debilitating conditions like epilepsy and multiple sclerosis. We will also discuss how marijuana has helped patients with conditions that are less common.

Reducing Problems Caused by Other Drugs

In some patients, marijuana can reduce the harsh symptoms brought about by other medical treatments. The best-known such use came with the advent of cancer chemotherapy. During chemotherapy, the body is infused with highly toxic substances, poisons designed to kill cancer cells. Unfortunately, those toxic substances produce many unwanted side-effects. We've all seen pictures of chemotherapy patients who have lost their hair. Less obvious, or rather less public, is the impact of chemotherapy on the digestive system.

Many patients on chemotherapy experience violent and extreme nausea. This is not the equivalent of getting carsick in the back seat, or even of that more extreme form of nausea, seasickness. Chemotherapy-induced nausea is far worse. One patient described it as a nuclear fire that would begin in her stomach and spread painfully throughout her body. Some doctors believe that as many as one in three chemotherapy patients discontinue their treatment because their nausea is unbearable. The risks associated with stopping treatment for a disease like cancer are all too obvious, but these patients feel they have no choice.

By now, tens of thousands of patients have learned that they can smoke a few puffs of marijuana prior to their chemotherapy treatments and eliminate this violent nausea – often with stunning success. Many believe that without marijuana they would be unable to continue the months of chemotherapy necessary to get results. When one hears a cancer chemotherapy patient state that marijuana saved his or her life, as many do, the claim often sounds preposterous. But it must be understood in the context of the severity of the nausea, the dramatic relief some patients have been able to achieve using marijuana, and the fact that such relief allows them to remain on the chemotherapy regime and ultimately conquer their cancer.

People with AIDS who are taking the new multi-drug 'cocktails' developed in the mid-1990s also often experience persistent and extreme nausea. The unpleasantness of such nausea, further complicated by the need to take dozens of pills each day, makes it difficult for many patients to stick with this very difficult regime. Failure to maintain all of the required dosages at regular intervals is, of course, life threatening. For many patients, marijuana can not only alleviate the nausea, but also help the patient maintain a normal appetite and thus remain strong and well-nourished during treatment.

Other medical patients experience less violent nausea but nausea that is nonetheless very debilitating. People with kidney failure who are on dialysis are an example of this. In these instances, the nausea is not life threatening, but it can severely disrupt a patient's ability to function, and it can lead to further complications.

Once again, keep in mind that the ability of marijuana to alleviate nausea in any disease situation will vary from person to person. Some will find that commercial antinausea medication works better than marijuana. For others, the opposite will be the case.

Treating Painful or Damaging Symptoms

Veterans Administration (VA) hospitals across the US care for numerous patients with spinal cord injuries received in Vietnam. Thanks to advances in helicopter design, for the first time in modern warfare, soldiers in Vietnam with these injuries could be airlifted directly off the battlefield to nearby hospitals. Whereas in past wars, such injuries frequently resulted in death, spinal cord damage during the Vietnam war often led instead to lifetime confinement in a wheelchair. Stroll through the paraplegic and quadriplegic wards in a typical VA hospital and you may often smell marijuana smoke.

The reason is that these patients often experience attacks of painful and uncontrollable muscle spasms. For many, marijuana has the ability to prevent these spasms. For others, marijuana is the most effective medicine with which to reduce the severity of the muscle contractions and the shakiness that often accompanies them.

Patients with multiple sclerosis also report fits of painful and uncontrollable muscle spasm (spasticity). Many of them have also become frequent marijuana users, as smoking marijuana seems to both alleviate and prevent this spasticity.

Glaucoma patients suffer from a condition in which pressure increases inside the eyeball. This eye pressure buildup occurs because blockage prevents the fluid inside the eyeball from draining out. As the pressure increases, it causes damage to parts of the retina. This in turn leads to partial, and sometimes complete, blindness. It is well known that smoking marijuana reduces internal eye pressure. Many glaucoma patients who use it report that their pain is reduced and their sight is improved. For some patients, marijuana use has become a daily activity they expect to continue throughout their lives. It is their way of preventing blindness.

Some patients who suffer from severe arthritic pain use marijuana as an analgesic (pain reliever), much as others of us use aspirin, paracetamol, ibuprofen or opiate-type narcotic pain relievers. They smoke marijuana on an as-needed basis to quell pain or to prevent pain from occurring at all.

As you can see, there is no single pattern for marijuana use. It depends on individual patients, specific conditions and current treatment goals. Marijuana is usually used on an as-needed basis, such as cancer chemotherapy treatment days. However, for some conditions, such as glaucoma, it may be necessary to use marijuana on a regular daily schedule and objectively measure eye pressures.

It is worth noting, also, that medical researchers are constantly developing new drugs to alleviate symptoms and reverse the conditions that create these many discomforts. Often they succeed. As an example, when the capacity of marijuana to lower intra-ocular (internal eye) pressure in glaucoma patients was first discovered, in the 1970s, there were very few other effective drugs on the market. Today, with newer glaucoma drugs available, marijuana may no longer be the most effective medication for many patients.

Enhancing and Restoring Normal Function

Marijuana can do more than relieve symptoms caused by other drugs, reduce pain, and treat uncomfortable or damaging conditions. For example, some patients with epilepsy or seizure disorders have problems not easily treatable. Major ('grand mal') epileptic seizures, the most severe kind, can deprive a person of bodily control and include convulsions, blackouts and loss of bladder and/or bowel control. The typical prescriptions for this disorder are nervous system depressants and muscle relaxants that often leave patients feeling groggy and disoriented. Increasingly, some epileptics are sharing stories of using marijuana to prevent such seizures. They find that daily marijuana use decreases the frequency or eliminates the seizures and leaves them with no unpleasant side-effects.

The most common effect of smoking marijuana is not only the mildly psychoactive high, but what marijuana users often call 'the munchies'. Marijuana makes you hungry. It produces a craving for food that many people satisfy by grabbing the nearest snack and munching away. For patients with AIDS, this aspect of marijuana sometimes saves lives. The later stages of AIDS are often accompanied by what is called the 'wasting syndrome', when patients lose their appetites and then their body weight. As a result of the wasting syndrome, they compromise their capacity to resist other diseases.

To reverse this so-called wasting syndrome, many patients with AIDS have begun to smoke marijuana for its well-known appetite-stimulating properties. This mysterious tendency of marijuana to dramatically increase hunger and create an intense desire for food has been the butt of much marijuana humour, but it has now entered the realm of medicine as a life-saving factor for some patients.

Dealing with Milder Symptoms

Marijuana can also be effective in treating milder symptoms. Its appetite-stimulating qualities are being noticed in the treatment of anorexia and bulimia. Its antinausea qualities are used to help people with mild or temporary nausea. Its pain-relieving qualities have helped women in many countries deal with menstrual cramps.

We haven't said anything yet about positive uses for marijuana's psychoactive properties. Many patients with acute or mild psychological symptoms also use marijuana. Some claim that occasional, or even frequent, marijuana smoking reduces stress. People prone to fits of rage claim marijuana 'balances' moods and reduces aggressive urges. Others claim marijuana lifts them out of depression, although there are also reports in the medical literature suggesting that marijuana can contribute to depression. Finally, many former alcohol and cocaine addicts report using marijuana as an effective substitute for such drug abuse.

As you can see, marijuana is many things to many people. Its impact varies from individual to individual. It is not a cure, but it can be a source of relief for a very wide range of symptoms. For many patients it is only a temporary expedient. For others, it quickly becomes an integral part of their lives.

Because a certain amount of legal jeopardy is involved in acquiring and using marijuana, it is always best to seek help from others. Share your marijuana experiments (therapeutic trials) with your doctor. As new medicines are developed, he or she can provide you with up-to-date information. Let your friends and family members know what you are doing. There is nothing to be ashamed of in using a medicine, legal or not, to alleviate a life-threatening or debilitating condition. Suffering alone always adds to a patient's difficulty. With the extra stress of using an illegal medicine, patients need all the support they can get.

Chapter 3

Why All the Controversy? What Does the Research Actually Show?

There is not a shred of scientific evidence that smoked marijuana is useful or needed.

— US Drug Tsar, Gen. Barry McCaffrey, 16 August 1996

Marijuana is the safest therapeutically active substance known to man . . . safer than many foods we commonly consume.

— US Judge Francis L. Young, 6 September 1988

The written record on medicinal marijuana stretches back over 2,000 years. Yet, after hundreds of studies, experiments and reports, there is still no consensus about its effects. Wildly emotional arguments rage about whether or not marijuana should be considered a legitimate medicine. Other than the opiate narcotics, it is hard to think of another medicinal plant that has generated so much worldwide controversy. With the experts unable to agree, it is understandable that patients are left wondering what to do.

Let's take a look at the history of this controversy, and then see if we can separate the scientific truth from the political distortion. You may be surprised to learn just how much time and energy has gone into this dispute, and how many countries and civilizations have been involved in it. It may also surprise you to learn that some of the most convincing scientific data supporting the medicinal use of marijuana has come from the very governments that now most vigorously oppose its use.

Ancient References to Marijuana as a Medicine

The most detailed ancient descriptions of the medicinal uses for marijuana come from China and India. Though modern high technology medicine does not commonly refer back to the medicinal practices of ancient civilizations, it is interesting to see to what extent marijuana was a fixture in some of their healing traditions. If nothing else, this confirms that marijuana has a significant medical history, and that modern claims for its medicinal uses have not been pulled from thin air.

The world's oldest surviving list of medical drugs is the Chinese *Shen-nung Pen-tshao Ching*, a pharmacopoeia compiled nearly 2,000 years ago. This book, which is based on oral traditions reaching back centuries more, gives marijuana the name 'ma'. The Chinese ideogram of 'ma' depicts two plants drying in the sunlight. The book lists more than 100 ailments treated with various parts of the marijuana plant. The smoking of marijuana seems to have been uncommon in ancient China. Instead, patients took it in liquid and food preparations, including extracts, and topical preparations.

The *Shen-nung* text specifically cites marijuana's value for reducing the pain of rheumatism (joint inflammation) and for treating digestive disorders, including constipation and diarrhoea. It is also recommended for use as an anaesthetic before surgical operations, and to ease the symptoms of patients with malaria and beriberi. Another Chinese text, written in 1578 by Li Shih Chen, also speaks of marijuana's use as an antinausea agent, an antibiotic and a means to stop haemorrhaging.

Literature from ancient India describes similar medical conditions for which various marijuana preparations were used. One commentator notes that marijuana 'has been intimately associated with magical, medical, religious and social customs in India for thousands of years.' Sushruta, an ancient Indian healer, recommended marijuana to relieve congestion and as part of a cure for fevers. Ayurveda, a traditional Hindu system of medicine practised in India since the first century AD, cites marijuana as an appetite stimulant, a digestive aid, a pain reliever and a sleeping potion.

In 1893, British colonial authorities decided to investigate the many uses of marijuana in India, in part as a scientific inquiry, and in part to determine the threat marijuana may have posed to the country. (Of course, the British didn't consider their own favourite intoxicant, alcohol, as a threat even though many of their Indian subjects most certainly did.) The investigation, conducted by the Indian Hemp Drugs Commission, heard testimony from Indian and Western doctors on the medical uses of marijuana. A wide range of claimed uses were discussed, including marijuana's ability to control spasms and cramps, to reduce pain, to fight digestive disorders, to anaesthetize patients facing minor surgery, and to ease asthma and bronchitis.

The British Commission was duly impressed. They took special note of the fact that many of the Indian medical applications of marijuana matched the way European doctors were utilizing the plant at the same time. In conclusion, the Commission wrote, '*Cannabis indica* (marijuana) must be looked upon as one of the most important drugs of Indian *Materia Medica* (their pharmacopoeia).'

There is ancient literature about marijuana from other parts of the world, as well, including Africa, the Middle East, ancient Greece and the Roman Empire. Like many modern references, these ancient descriptions of how marijuana is used in disease treatment also mention the psychological effects of the drug, but in these cases it is often in glowing terms. These texts credit marijuana with quickening the mind, enhancing concentration, eliminating stress, creating joyful feelings and enhancing sexual pleasure. The fact that marijuana had medical value was never very far removed from the fact that it also made people feel good.

Marijuana Is Outlawed in America – over Doctors' Objections

Marijuana products were in widespread use in the United States during the 19th century. Doctors recommended marijuana to treat a variety of ailments and pharmacists sold marijuana over-the-counter as an ingredient in numerous remedies. However, marijuana began to lose its role in medicine with the development of aspirin, which displaced it as a routine painkiller. When opium-derived drugs such as morphine found increasing use in surgery and other medical applications, the popularity of marijuana declined further.

During the period of Prohibition of Alcohol (1920–1933), the psychoactive properties of marijuana left it open to criticism by some of the same moralistic and religious forces who opposed consumption of the psychoactive drug, alcohol. Eventually, these forces prevailed. In 1937, Congress passed the Marijuana Tax Act which effectively made continued use of marijuana a criminal offence.

During hearings conducted before the passage of the Marijuana Tax Act, the lone opponent was a representative of the American Medical Association (AMA). He was treated derisively by committee members who questioned why the medical profession had not been more aggressive in fighting the 'menace' of marijuana. Nonetheless, the AMA representative argued that any law banning marijuana should at least exempt it for medical purposes. His testimony included this statement:

> There is positively no evidence to indicate the abuse of cannabis (marijuana) as a medicinal agent or to show that its medicinal use is leading to the development of cannabis addiction. Cannabis at the present time is slightly used for medicinal purposes, but it would seem worthwhile to maintain its status as a medicinal agent . . . There is a possibility that a restudy of the drug by modern means may show other advantages to be derived from its medicinal use.

Over AMA objections, marijuana was removed from the American pharmacopoeia in 1941, and any hope for further research or legal medical use of marijuana came to an end. In 1970, Congress restructured federal drug laws with the Controlled Substances Act, which repeated the initial mistake and kept marijuana banned for medicinal use.

Marijuana Is Outlawed in the UK

Cannabis became illegal in the UK after the country agreed to the 1925 Geneva International Convention on Narcotics Control. It was included in the Convention under proposals by the Egyptians and the Turks. An Egyptian delegate announced that 'chronic hashism' has caused most of the insanity in his country. It also, he said, weakened users, gave them heart and digestive troubles and made them look wild-eyed and stupid.

India opposed including cannabis in the Convention, as their delegate said it had been used there since time immemorial, grew wild and they doubted that a prohibition could be enforced. The British delegate abstained from the vote but signed in the end. There was hardly any parliamentary debate before it came into law as amendments to the Dangerous Drugs Act on 28 September 1928.

Despite this, cannabis convictions were minor, and the drug was still used medicinally as required. Such were the societal pressures to legalize marijuana in the 1960s, that the Home Office initiated a report into the drug's effects. Chaired by Baroness Wootton, the Select Committee recommended that possession should no longer be regarded as a serious crime and imprisonment should no longer be viewed as an appropriate penalty in cases of possession.

By the time the Wootton report came out, the Conservatives had lost the election, and the new Labour government totally rejected the Wootton recommendations. In 1971, the Home Secretary introduced the Misuse of Drugs Act, which remains in force today. Although opiates and other narcotics were still used in medicine, cannabis was banned, largely because inadequate research into its effects had taken place.

Modern Research on Medical Marijuana Begins

Just after passage of the Controlled Substances Act in the US, the first new, modern medical use for the drug was discovered. In a strange bit of irony, a UCLA researcher began a study to develop methods by which the police could detect whether or not a person was intoxicated with marijuana. Instead, he inadvertently discovered marijuana's ability to reduce intra-ocular (internal eye) pressure and help patients with glaucoma. The researcher had intended to assess whether or not the pupil dilation that often accompanies marijuana smoking could be used by police to tell who was high and who was not. But he stumbled on a finding that saved many glaucoma patients from blindness, and led to a new area of medical research.

Soon after, when cancer chemotherapy was in its early stages and the substances used were highly toxic, word began to spread among patients that marijuana could eliminate the intense nausea that many experienced during treatment. During this period, in the early 1970s, the social and cultural changes provoked by the movements of the 1960s had led to the widespread recreational use of marijuana. Some cancer patients were also recreational users, and they discovered, by accident, that their recreational use of marijuana reduced chemotherapy-induced nausea.

Something similar was happening in America's Veterans Administration hospitals. US troops in Vietnam had easy access to large quantities of marijuana. Many became frequent recreational users. Some of these soldiers received spinal cord injuries and continued their recreational marijuana use. These disabled veterans discovered that marijuana could control the painful muscle spasms associated with spinal cord injury.

Synthetic THC (Marinol)

During this period, scientists discovered the principal psychoactive ingredient in marijuana, delta-9-tetrahydrocannabinol (delta-9-THC or just THC). This was the compound primarily responsible for the psychoactive condition or high associated with marijuana use. Later research revealed that the high probably resulted from a complex interaction of several compounds in marijuana, but there is no doubt that THC is the principal cause.

At this point, modern medicine had what it needed to partially accept marijuana – a single synthetic chemical compound that could be isolated, patented, manufactured and distributed for profit by a drug company. THC was tested and found to relieve the nausea caused by cancer chemotherapy. In the US, the FDA approved it for sale for that purpose, and later for AIDS wasting syndrome, and it was put on the market under the brand name, Marinol.®

Nevertheless, concentrated THC was a powerful psychoactive drug and many patients didn't like it. They complained that it made them too high (a condition called dysphoria), or that it caused intense anxiety, or that it kept them from carrying on normal activities for up to six hours at a time. In the US, patients also complained about the price of Marinol. A year's supply can cost as much as $15,000, too high a price to pay, some said, for a flawed version of a common weed easily grown in anyone's backyard. There were many other complaints about Marinol, as well.

Patients experiencing extreme nausea find it difficult to swallow any medication in pill form. Some patients vomit when trying to swallow the capsule and are unable to use it. When Marinol does work, many patients claim it takes over an hour to relieve their symptoms. This probably results from the fact that the THC passes through the liver before reaching the receptors in the brain where psychoactive reactions and nausea suppressions take place. Because Marinol takes so long to reduce nausea, some patients have complained that they are at risk of overdosing when they are driven to get quick relief from their violent symptoms.

One of the reasons many patients prefer smoking marijuana to swallowing Marinol is that it allows them to regulate precisely the amount of THC they take into their systems. Because smoking permits an almost instantaneous transmission of the THC in the marijuana to sites in the brain where it works to control nausea, patients are able to simply continue smoking until the nausea subsides. This allows some to stop smoking before they get high. When the antinausea effect wears off, they can smoke a little more if they need to. Since individuals respond differently to different doses, smoking allows patients to determine the proper dose for themselves. As a result, they can avoid taking too much, which is not possible with Marinol.

It has been suggested by researchers that cannabidiol, one of the 460 known compounds in marijuana smoke, actually reduces some of the anxiety brought on by THC in its pure form (Grinspoon, 1997; 44). While some patients report feelings of anxiety or discomfort after using either drug, these feelings generally cease to occur in those who repeatedly administer smoked marijuana. Patients who were unfamiliar with smoked marijuana initially, describe more pleasurable feelings after they are acquainted with, and can anticipate, its effects. With Marinol, on the other hand, many patients report that it has an unpleasant and debilitating effect on them even with continued use.

While most patients seem to prefer smoked marijuana to Marinol, some prefer Marinol or marijuana ingested in food because of a general aversion to smoking. This is the most common concern voiced about smoking marijuana instead of ingesting it. Some patients who prefer marijuana instead of Marinol, but do not like to smoke, choose to cook the marijuana into food. Baked brownies are the most popular way to do this. Marijuana can also be added to alcohol, oil or butter, and it can be used to make beverages, sauces and other baked foods. There are many methods of administering medicinal marijuana; however, patients using it to combat nausea generally do not want to eat anything to gain relief. Eating marijuana in any form has many of the same problems of delay and dose control that THC does.

British Cannabis

Marinol, also known as Dronabinol, is not licensed in the UK, although it may be in the future. At present, the only licensed cannabinoid is Nabilone, marketed under the trade name Cesamet.

Nabilone is a synthetic cannabinoid with anti-emetic properties which have been found to be of value in the management of some patients with nausea and vomiting associated with cancer chemotherapy. It also has sedative and psychotropic effects. The manufacturers warn that Nabilone should be used with extreme caution in patients with severe liver dysfunction and in those with a history of non-psychotic emotional disorders. Nabilone should not be taken with alcohol, sedatives, hypnotics or other psychotomimetic substances. Since Nabilone will often impair the mental and/or physical abilities required for the performance of potentially hazardous tasks, such as driving a car and operating machinery, the patient should be warned accordingly and should not be permitted to drive or engage in dangerous tasks until the effects of Nabilone are no longer present. Adverse psychiatric reactions can persist for 48 to 72 hours following cessation of treatment.

Since Nabilone elevates supine and standing heart rates and causes postural hypotension, it should be used with caution in the elderly and in patients with hypertension or heart disease.

The most frequently observed adverse reactions to Nabilone reported in the course of clinical trials were as follows: drowsiness, vertigo, psychological high, dry mouth, depression, ataxia, blurred vision, sensation disturbance, anorexia, headache, orthostatic hypotension, euphoria and hallucinations. The following adverse reactions were observed in less than 1 per cent of the patients who were administered Nabilone in the course of the clinical trials: tachycardia, tremors, syncope, nightmares, distortion in the perception of time, confusion, dissociation, dysphoria, psychotic reactions and seizures.

Interestingly, the range of side-effects experienced with Nabilone is far greater than it is for using the marijuana plant in its entirety. Indeed, some of the side-effects of Nabilone are precisely those symptoms that marijuana is believed to ease, including anorexia and depression.

Nabilone was first licensed in the 1970s, following the criminalization of marijuana, and is licensed as an anti-emetic in chemotherapy treatments. Its indications are, precisely, 'for the control of nausea and vomiting caused by chemotherapeutic agents in the treatment of cancer in patients who have failed to respond adequately to conventional anti-emetic methods'. According to the manufacturer, the beneficial effects of cannabis, for example, in relieving the painful effects of muscle spasticity in MS, are 'entirely anecdotal', although they concede that the clinical trials under way in the UK at present are set up to evaluate scientifically just that.

Under the strict UK regulatory system, a doctor may prescribe either an unlicensed medicine or a medicine that is licensed but for a different indication to that for which he is prescribing. Theoretically, doctors could prescribe Dronabinol (as Marinol), which is currently licensed in the USA only, and there is some evidence to suggest that they do. However, if a doctor does prescribe either Marinol or Cesamet for any condition other than nausea and vomiting caused by chemotherapy, he or she takes full responsibility for the use of the product. The mechanism is known as a 'Named Patient

Prescription'. Such prescriptions are executed under strict controls, and the doctor must keep accurate records of the patient and the product.

The patient will then take his prescription to the pharmacist. In the case of Nabilone, the pharmacist must contact Cambridge Laboratories (the manufacturer) to place an order. Cambridge Laboratories will require the name and address of the prescribing doctor and an assurance that a record is made of the patient's name before the product can be dispatched. Cambridge Laboratories have accurate records of each transaction, and these records are subject to random inspection by the Medicines Control Agency.

The current cost of Nabilone is £110 for 20 tablets, and recommended dosage is between 1 and 6 mg daily. Twenty tablets, therefore, could last between 4 and 20 days, depending on the severity of the condition treated. The cost of this medicine to the health service roughly equates to the cost of Marinol to the individual in the US. Marijuana could be provided for less than one-tenth of the cost, and probably even less.

State-Sponsored Research on Marijuana in America

As interest in marijuana for medical applications grew, scientists undertook new research studies. Simultaneously, a minor public outcry erupted over the injustice of sending seriously, even terminally, ill patients to jail for marijuana violations. Many patients bravely defended their marijuana use in public and pleaded with elected officials to change the laws that branded them as criminals.

New Mexico launched the first official state-sponsored

marijuana research programme. Five other states eventually followed suit, including California, New York, Tennessee, Michigan and Georgia. Each of these state studies relied on marijuana supplied by the US government, and the research designs were all approved by the Food and Drug Administration.

The report on New Mexico's research programme (Dansak, 1986) that was conducted from 1979 to 1986 stated that marijuana was not only effective as an antinausea drug, but also that it was 'far superior to the best available conventional drug, Compazine [Buccastem or Stemetil in the UK], and clearly superior to the synthetic THC pill.' The study, which reported on 169 patients, found that 'more than 90 per cent of the patients who received marijuana . . . reported significant or total relief from nausea and vomiting,' with no major side-effects (Randall, 1990; 149). All the patients in the study had to prove, as a condition of participation, that they had tried other antinausea drugs without success.

In the New York state research programme, 199 patients suffering from nausea induced by cancer chemotherapy were given marijuana between 1982 and 1985. Over 90 per cent reported it to be effective in reducing their symptoms (Vinciguerra, 1988). The California state research programme was much larger, involving thousands of patients between 1981 and 1989. Like the New Mexico programme, THC and smoked marijuana were both part of the California research protocol. By 1983, their annual report concluded, 'The California Program also has met its research objectives. Marijuana has been shown to be effective for many cancer chemotherapy patients, safe dosage levels have been established, and a dosage regimen which minimizes undesirable side effects has been devised and tested (Randall, 1990; 235).'

Even the US government found some merit in the medical

use of marijuana. In 1976, a glaucoma patient in Washington, DC, was arrested for growing a small amount of marijuana. When he was charged with illegal cultivation, he raised a 'medical necessity' defence and was acquitted. An agency of the government decided to resolve this contradiction in the law by supplying the patient with marijuana. This 'solution' allowed him to avoid illegally growing it himself, or illegally purchasing it from others. The government was willing to look the other way with respect to the illegality of his possession of marijuana.

Over the next 14 years, the US government approved marijuana distribution to a handful of other patients. Then, in 1990, they were deluged with about 400 new applications, mostly from patients with AIDS who were beginning to discover that marijuana could benefit them, as well. About two dozen of these applications were approved before officials suddenly discontinued the programme in 1992. In all, some 34 patients were at one time receiving marijuana from the government. Eight of those patients survive today.

Nothing reveals the contradictions in US policy towards marijuana more clearly than the fact that there are still eight patients in the United States who receive a tin of marijuana 'joints' (cigarettes) every month from the government. The marijuana is grown for the government on a small plot administered by the University of Mississippi. These eight people can legally possess and use marijuana, at government expense and with government permission. Yet hundreds of thousands of other patients can be fined and jailed under federal law for doing exactly the same thing.

An objective observer might have concluded that with the findings coming out of the various state research programmes, and the government's unwillingness to help at least a few patients, laws regarding the medical use of marijuana would have been relaxed by the early 1980s. Unfortunately, that period coincided with widespread national concern over illegal drug use, most of it involving heroin, crack cocaine and other hard drugs. First Lady Nancy Reagan launched her 'Just Say No' campaign, and her husband's administration dramatically increased penalties and enforcement appropriations for drug offences.

Marijuana, a soft drug, was lumped in with the others because of the mistaken belief that it led, almost inevitably, to hard drug use. Once that happened, any hope of a special dispensation for the medical use of marijuana was lost, captive of the new political realities. Equally tragic, all research on the medical uses of marijuana came to a screeching halt, since the only legal source for marijuana was the federal farm in Mississippi, and officials stopped making any of their crop available to scientists.

Politics Triggers Renewed Interest in Marijuana Research

Politics, once responsible for blocking medical marijuana research, has more recently been the source of renewed interest in it. The passage of California's Proposition 215 in November 1996, which permitted patients to use marijuana under state law, created a national political earthquake. Contradictions in government policy were exposed to millions, and quickly turned a majority of Americans against laws that prevented patients from using marijuana. A national poll conducted by ABC-TV and the Discovery Channel six months later revealed that 69 per cent of the American people favoured the legalization of marijuana for medical use. This situation is echoed in the UK. In 1998, BBC's *Healthcheck* ran a telephone poll, asking viewers whether they believed cannabis should be legalized for medical purposes. An astonishing 96 per cent said yes, while only 4 per cent believed that cannabis should remain illegal. A *Disability Now* survey found much the same results. Their survey of disabled people showed that 195 out of 200 disabled people questioned believed that it should be legalized.

With public opinions swinging so dramatically against them, American government officials were forced to moderate their policies. Their basic opposition to medical marijuana did not change. What did change was their public attitude towards research. Various promises were made that scientists would once again be permitted to conduct research and that federally grown marijuana would be supplied to them under tightly controlled conditions. But as of this writing, at the end of 1997, only one scientist in the entire nation has actually received permission to go forward. Hopefully, he will soon be joined by others.

Unlike the environment faced by researchers and the patients in 1970s and early 1980s, medical marijuana research today would be conducted under the spotlight of the mass media, with an active national political controversy brewing in the background. Voters in several states are likely to be considering ballot initiatives in 1998 similar to Proposition 215 in California. Hopefully, political efforts of this sort, alongside ongoing research work, will lead to a resolution of the medical marijuana controversy that is based on science instead of politics.

UK Change of Heart

The UK situation is looking less bleak. The unquestionable public support for the legalization of cannabis for medicinal purposes has, along with the support for a number of MPs and lobby groups, including Alliance for Cannabis Therapeutics (ACT) and *Disability Now*, convinced the British government that the time has come to rethink policy.

Just two years ago, no clinical studies were being made into the benefit of cannabis for medicinal purposes, despite Home Secretary Jack Straw's assurances that some were ongoing. Speaking on Radio Four's *Today* programme, Mr Straw said, 'There is no reason why cannabis should not be available for medicinal purposes if people can prove that it has therapeutic effect.' He called on doctors and pharmaceutical firms to get licences for research projects (a previously difficult proposition) and said that there were currently 19 licences issued by the Home Office. However, research by the BBC revealed that only six licences existed to look into the medicinal use. Three were found to have already lapsed, one was still current but no work was going on, and the other two were only testing cannabis compounds.

The British Medical Association (BMA) spoke out, and claimed that it wants to set up a research group to speed up studies into the effects of cannabis-based products. Head of Science and Ethics at the BMA, Dr Vivienne Nathanson, said, 'We want high quality research. We think this group will encourage people to put forward good projects and help liaise with the Home Office to minimize delay in approving new rules.'

In response the government granted a licence for cannabis to be grown for research purposes, and the House of Lords joined in the debate. At least 228 MPs and members of the House of Lords in the All Party Disablement Group backed *Disability Now*'s survey, which found that 97 per cent of readers thought that cannabis should be legalized as medicine. The British Medical Association called for the Misuse of Drugs Act to be amended so that prescribing certain extracts of the cannabis plant would no longer be illegal. In its report, 'Therapeutic Uses of Cannabis', it urges the use of a central registry of patients using extracts, and more tests on 'the remarkably safe drugs', which it says have fewer side-effects than some stronger, legal drugs.

The campaign was spearheaded by MPs Paul Flynn and Clare Short, whose fight centres around the fact that marijuana has been proven safe and effective for a wide range of illnesses. The House of Commons took note.

In late 1998, GW Pharmaceuticals was given the go-ahead by the Home Office to grow thousands of cannabis plants at a secret government-approved farm. The Home Office granted two licences; one is a cultivation licence allowing the company to grow cannabis, and the other allows the possession and supply of cannabis for medical research. GW Pharmaceuticals is collaborating with Dutch medicinal cannabis breeding specialists HortaPharm BV, which has extensive experience in cultivating cannabis for medical purposes.

An initial crop of 5000 plants was sown in August 1998 in a glasshouse in the south of England. Eventually 20,000 plants will be cultivated at the facility. Dr Geoffrey Guy, chairman of GW Pharmaceuticals, said, 'The potential benefits of cannabis are absolutely enormous. We are only beginning to take the blinders off that have been on this material for the last 30 years.' Dr Guy said the first aim of his research would be to establish a safe dose to give to patients that would reproduce the medical benefits without the 'high' associated with the recreational use of the drug. Once that had been established, the drug would be tested for its ability to relieve the pain associated with nerve damage in conditions such as multiple sclerosis, spina bifida and spinal cord injuries. Dr Guy also intends to test the impact of cannabis on minimizing brain injuries suffered by stroke victims, and its ability to improve sight and hearing in the deaf and blind.

In early 1999, two doctors volunteered to begin the first official trials for the therapeutic use of cannabis. Dr Anita Holdcroft from the Hammersmith Hospital in London will test whether cannabis or its active components can be used to relieve post-operative pain. Three hundred patients will take part.

Dr John Zajicek of Derriford Hospital in Plymouth will begin a trial of 600 patients into whether cannabis is effective in treating muscular rigidity in multiple sclerosis sufferers. Experts from the Royal Pharmaceutical Society (RPS) and the Medical Research Council published protocols on how to carry out legal trials on cannabis.

If the results of the trials are accepted by the World Health Organization, they could lead to the UK government legalizing cannabis for medical use. It is expected that it will take at least six months for the trials to be set up, but if they prove that the drug is beneficial, named patients could be prescribed the drug within three years. Under the present protocols, only people with multiple sclerosis and post-operative pain will be able to have marijuana on prescription, if the studies are successful. However, it does open the door to further research.

A recent House of Lords Science and Technology Committee report backed the studies. It stated that while the House believed that the recreational use of cannabis should remain illegal, they proposed listing cannabis as a 'schedule two' drug, downgrading it from its current prohibited 'schedule one' status. The government called for more clinical trials before a change in the drug laws could be considered.

Anecdotal Evidence vs. Controlled Scientific Research

Before leaving the subject of scientific research, a final comment is necessary regarding the reliability of medical claims for marijuana. Research findings on marijuana have been criticized for being unscientific or anecdotal. There is a kernel of truth in these claims. Marijuana research cannot easily be fitted into the typical model of a controlled scientific study because it simply isn't possible to create an effective placebo for marijuana.

Rigorously controlled studies on marijuana with human subjects would require the formation of two groups, only one of which receives marijuana. The other, or control, group would get a placebo, a substance outwardly identical to marijuana but with none of its telltale qualities. If members of the two groups have been selected at random, and if the groups are sufficiently large, differences between the two groups can be attributed to the presence or absence of marijuana.

Unfortunately, the psychoactive properties of marijuana make it impossible to create a placebo. A researcher can give a subject something to smoke that looks and even smells like marijuana. It is called hemp, marijuana's nonpsychoactive cousin. Hemp is a plant used to make rope, cloth and paper. It is very similar to marijuana, but has no psychoactive properties. Just like marijuana, growing or possessing raw hemp is illegal in the United States. In the UK, the Home Office allowed the relaxation of restrictions concerning hemp in 1993, albeit under strict licensing controls. Despite its outward similarity to marijuana, anyone smoking industrial hemp will instantly know that it is not marijuana precisely because it doesn't have those psychoactive properties that are instantly evident with marijuana.

Therefore, marijuana can never be researched in tightly controlled scientific studies. That does not mean that all research on marijuana is invalid. The New Mexico state study, cited above, allowed people to compare marijuana versus oral THC (Marinol) or the UK-licensed cannabinoid, Nabilone, with respect to the ability of each to control nausea. The subjects then reported to the researchers which substances worked best. Instead of accepting such research as valid, some scientific critics of medical marijuana take the very orthodox position that the self-reports of the subjects are not reliable. They argue that such reports are possibly coloured by what the subjects want to believe.

Certainly, this is possible. But when study after study yields similar results, when those results are supported by decades, if not centuries, of similar experience, it is time for medical marijuana opponents to concede that the research conclusions have some validity. These results are valid even though they are often based on patient's subjective (anecdotal) responses rather than objective measurements by the researchers. Furthermore, when the substance in question has been in worldwide use for millennia and has been conclusively demonstrated to pose no threat to life or limb, it is simply cruel not to allow patients to derive what benefit they can from it.

The term 'anecdotal evidence' is a pejorative one in science. It is used to put down nonrigorous research. But when hundreds, thousands, even tens of thousands of patients come forward, all describing the same phenomenon in more or less the same terms, it is time to put scientific rigours aside and accept the obvious truth. Certainly, that has happened regarding marijuana's ability to alleviate nausea, to stimulate appetite, and to control muscle spasms. It is beginning to happen in a host of other areas, as well, as the next chapters in this book will demonstrate.

Many doctors care for patients on a daily basis in clinics, offices and hospitals. These 'clinical' doctors often have different attitudes than doctors who concentrate primarily on research. Good clinical doctors seek anecdotal evidence from patients to help with diagnosis and treatment. This is especially true when managing subjective problems such as nausea and pain. It would be impossible to evaluate an antinausea or antipain medication without the use of important subjective anecdotal evidence. Listening to anecdotal evidence over many years transmits valuable education to doctors and contributes to clinical experience. One of us (RB) went to a medical school where the motto was 'The patient is the textbook'. Clinical experience and academic research are both important in providing optimal medical care.

Additional research is always welcome. Using the lack of controlled studies to forestall acceptance of the medicinal uses of marijuana, particularly for extraneous political, moral or religious reasons, can no longer be justified. Penicillin was first put on the market after being tested on only six human subjects, hardly enough to qualify as a scientifically rigorous test. However, to withhold penicillin after seeing what it did for those six patients would have been a criminal act, given what it could do for everyone else.

Chapter 4
Nausea and Cancer Chemotherapy

In the United States and the United Kingdom today, the most common medicinal use of marijuana is as an anti-emetic, the technical name for a substance that reduces nausea and vomiting. The largest patient population using it for that purpose is people with cancer who are being treated with chemotherapy or radiation. Such treatment involves very unpleasant side-effects that can last for hours, days or even weeks. At times, these side-effects can be more distressing and debilitating than the cancer itself. The nausea can be so severe that a patient will spend hours vomiting or dry heaving. Some patients have even broken or fractured bones in the process.

Not surprisingly, many chemotherapy and radiation patients lose their appetites. So severe is the nausea that some are unable to eat or even tolerate the smell of food. They lose weight rapidly, which contributes to their physical deterioration, and even to their premature death. Others become so fearful of having to repeat the experience that they reject further treatment, a desperate choice that exposes them to increased risk and premature death from their cancers.

If you have been diagnosed with cancer, you will face many choices about your treatment. Depending upon your condition and the opinion of your doctor, you may or may not choose to combat your illness with chemotherapy, and it may or may not work for you. Whatever your own decision, you should know that there are other people who have chosen chemotherapy and feel that, in spite of the grave side-effects, it prolonged or saved their lives. Many such people will tell you that chemotherapy worked for them because they found a way to tolerate its side-effects. Some did this through standard prescription drugs. Others succeeded only with marijuana, either with or without the approval and guidance of their doctors.

A number of drugs are routinely prescribed to treat the side-effects of anticancer chemotherapy. Drugs to treat nausea and vomiting include Ativan, Buccastem, Stemetil, Kytril, Phenergan, Prozière, Avomine, Cinaziere, Stugeron, Motilium, hyoscine and Dramamine. No doubt, your doctor will prescribe the one most likely to help you. If it fails to provide you with the relief you want and need, there will be others to try, as well. Eventually, your doctor may suggest that you try Marinol (Dronabinol) or Cesamet (Nabilone). This is the synthetic chemical delta-9-tetrahydrocannabinol, or THC, that is one of the active ingredients in marijuana.

Marinol and Cesamet are promoted as safer and more effective than marijuana, because it is manufactured under controlled conditions, can be dispensed in precise doses and is pharmaceutically pure. Marinol works for some patients but doesn't work well for others. As we said in Chapter 3, THC (Marinol) is a powerful psychoactive drug. Patients sometimes complain that it makes them too high, causes anxiety and/or prevents them from carrying on normal activities. Patients with nausea and vomiting often can't swallow a pill to get relief. There are other complaints about Marinol. It is often too slow to take effect. It is very expensive. In addition, like other antinausea drugs, it sometimes loses its effectiveness over periods of prolonged use. Given the options available, thousands of patients are choosing to treat themselves with marijuana, and many of them are doing so with the tacit approval of their doctors.

The use of marijuana as an antinausea medication was rediscovered by modern medicine in the early 1970s, around the same time that the use of chemotherapy in cancer treatment was becoming widespread. Some young cancer patients, like so many other young people at the time, were experimenting with marijuana. They brought its antinausea capability to the attention of doctors. American psychiatrist and author Dr Lester Grinspoon was among the first to advocate the use of marijuana as a medicine. In 1971, Dr Grinspoon's own teenage son, Danny, was getting chemotherapy for leukaemia. Danny, who had never used marijuana for recreational purposes, was having severe side-effects of nausea, vomiting and anorexia. When Danny became discouraged from the side-effects, he begged his parents to quit the chemotherapy.

At a dinner party for a Harvard doctor, Danny's mother listened as Dr Emil Frei discussed anecdotal cases of how marijuana reduced chemotherapy side-effects. In compassionate disregard for the law, Danny's mother illegally obtained marijuana for her dying son. Danny smoked marijuana before chemotherapy treatments to prevent his nausea and vomiting and quickly discovered he could now eat. He also agreed to continue chemotherapy once his side-effects from treatment were controlled. This allowed Danny to spend an additional year with his family and friends before he died (Randall, 1990; 5–7). The first clinical study on the use of marijuana in chemotherapy was conducted shortly thereafter. Other doctors at Harvard soon became aware that some patients were successfully using marijuana, not only to relieve their nausea, but also to regain their appetites.

While it is not common for patients to lead doctors to new

methods of treatment, it is not as uncommon as you might think. Some folk remedies have been used to treat patients in modern clinical trials. On occasion, these remedies are found to work. When doctors first observed that marijuana could effectively control nausea and vomiting, they set up clinical trials to test their observations.

Doctors Sallan and Zinberg from Harvard were among the first to report the positive benefits of oral THC to control chemotherapy-induced nausea and vomiting (Sallan, 1975). Of significant interest is that ten to twelve patients dropped out of the study because smoked marijuana was more effective. The National Cancer Institute conducted a pivotal study in 1979 that showed that the effectiveness of oral THC and smoked marijuana was related to the blood concentration of THC. In other words, the higher the concentration of THC, the greater the benefit. They found inhaled marijuana to be more effective (Chang, 1979).

During this same time, cancer patients and their physicians across the United States pushed to make marijuana available for medical use. In New Mexico, one indefatigable cancer patient, Lynn Pierson, struggled to implement a study to compare oral THC to smoked marijuana. It concluded that inhaled marijuana was more effective than oral THC in decreasing the severity of nausea and vomiting (Dansak, 1986).

In New York state, cancer patients who had failed to get relief with standard antinausea drugs and oral THC were supplied with marijuana cigarettes and 78 per cent of these patients benefited from the inhaled marijuana (Vinciguerra, 1988). The Department of Public Health in Michigan initiated a study in 1979 to compare Torecan (a commonly prescribed drug that counters nausea) to inhaled marijuana. Participants could elect to switch from the assigned drug to the alternative. The results were statistically equal. However, greater than 90 per cent of patients receiving Torecan elected to try marijuana and 90 per cent of patients using marijuana did not elect to switch. Studies done in California and Tennessee also proved the effectiveness of oral THC and smoked marijuana to reduce the nausea and vomiting caused by cancer chemotherapy (Randall, 1990; 234). As a result, patients and their doctors became aware of the benefits of smoked marijuana to manage the side-effects of cancer chemotherapy.

One such patient was Jo Daly, a former police commissioner in San Francisco, California. She used marijuana in 1988 to survive chemotherapy for cancer of the colon, and again in 1995, when doctors found a malignant tumour in her left lung. In the following address to the citizens of San Francisco, and to the San Francisco Board of Supervisors, she explained the circumstances that led to her use of marijuana:

> My name is Jo Daly. In May of 1988, I was discovered to have cancer of the colon, phase IV, which had metastasized. Emergency surgery took my ovaries, my uterus, part of my colon and some lymph nodes. Six months of chemotherapy followed.
>
> About five hours after completing my very first treatment, I felt a fever rise, all over. Before I could even take my temperature, what can only be described as a nuclear implosion occurred. Centered in my solar plexus, an incredible heat radiated and blasted throughout my limbs. Even my fingernails and toenails burned. Then the nausea began in earnest, lasting three solid hours, leaving me helplessly weak. Needless to say, I didn't have much of an appetite and, though physically exhausted, I could hardly sleep that night. I was anticipating the repeat therapy that awaited me the next morning. And the morning after that. And the morning after that.

The next day, I prepared myself by taking Compazine (Stemetil or Buccastem) before leaving the house. I was administered Ativan at the clinic, and I'd even left out a Marinol gel cap by my bed. Home, after the treatment, I meditated for relaxation and listened to a positive imagery exercise in order to take mental control of the situation. But a few hours later, I sensed the emerging fever again, grabbed the Marinol and swallowed it. Back came the nausea and the nuclear implosion burning throughout my body. Once again, I was reduced to a kneeling position over the toilet for another three hours. It felt like three years.

On the third day of my treatment, I took the Compazine, and was given an Ativan (lorazepam), and submitted once more to the poison. Once again, about five hours after returning home from the clinic, that familiar fever began its emergence. This time I closed the door to my room and lit up a marijuana cigarette that had been given to me by a friend. I took three puffs and put it out. I sat quietly and meditated, advising my body to relax, telling myself that it would be OK this time. Within a half an hour, the fever subsided. No nuclear implosion took place, no vomiting, very minor nausea – and I actually ate a sandwich later on that evening. I slept well for the first time since I could remember.

I won't say the next six months were bliss. But I got through them by using marijuana. And my doctor approved. Another patient provided me the phone number of an underground source of marijuana, just for legitimate patients. No charge – but those who could afford it made a donation. Not wishing to smoke, I found that a marijuana cookie or brownie could last me three or four days of treatments. I tried the Marinol several times again, but it simply didn't work. Since I never possessed more than a little marijuana at a time, I knew that under our city policy, the worst that could happen would be that I'd get a citation and a $100 fine, rather than be taken to jail. Still, breaking the law, however minor, created stress. And stress is known to interfere with healing. But I needed the chemotherapy in order to survive. And I needed the marijuana in order to survive the chemotherapy.

Sadly, Jo Daly passed away in 1997. Another woman from San Francisco, Judith Cushner, had much better luck. Judith, 52, is the mother of two young adult children. She is the administrator of a preschool. In 1990, after being diagnosed with breast cancer, she used marijuana to survive seven months of chemotherapy and radiation treatment. She began using marijuana on the advice of a paediatric oncology nurse. She has been cancer free since her last treatment in November, 1990.

I was diagnosed with breast cancer at the age of 45, on my daughter's 13th birthday. My doctors found a very small but virulent tumor during a routine mammogram. They thought it should be treated aggressively because of my age. Over the next seven months, I underwent eight rounds of chemotherapy and radiation, immediately following a lumpectomy to remove the tumor.

I started my chemotherapy taking three of the standard drugs at the time, in combination. I took two of them intravenously, every other week. The third, called Cytoxan (Endoxana), I took orally every day. Cytoxan, I have learned, is a drug that was developed from nerve gas during the World War II. When I was taking it, I experienced constant nausea. It wasn't as violent as the nausea I would get immediately after taking the intravenous drugs, but it lingered with me night and day, throwing off my balance, and killing my appetite. Sometimes, just looking at the bottle could make me feel sick. My oncologist advised me to take it at night, just before bed, so that its metabolic action could occur when I didn't need to be productive. As a result, I could never sleep very well.

Following my second round of chemotherapy, I experienced even more severe nausea. Within a few hours, I began dry heaving and I wasn't able to stand up. My doctor gave me a common antinausea drug called Compazine (Stemetil), to which I had an allergic reaction. Not only was I still feeling nauseous, but I started to feel as if I was crawling out of my own skin. All my nerve endings were inflamed, and I became almost completely immobilized.

I stopped taking the Compazine, and my doctor grew worried because I wasn't eating. So he took me off the Cytoxan, which was the most highly toxic of my treatments, and he put me on another intravenous drug instead. Then we discussed my need for a more effective antinausea drug in order to continue my therapy.

In the course of the conversation he brought up Marinol, but he said that it hadn't proven to be very effective for people in my age group. He also said that it didn't have the same effect as marijuana. I thought that what he said was a little curious, but I took a prescription for Marinol. I had to go to three pharmacies before I could get it filled, given that it is such a highly controlled substance.

Unfortunately the Marinol didn't work so well, either. The capsules were like those huge, oily vitamins, and they were extremely difficult to take. They weren't doing much for my nausea, and they made me very sleepy, so I couldn't function on them. I was already stressed about losing my everyday abilities and not being there for my children. I felt like I was going to be that way every day for an eternity, and it depressed me. Every Saturday morning, the morning after my treatments, I experienced constant retching, going from the bedroom to the bathroom without stopping.

At the time, I had chosen to go in for my treatments on Friday evenings because that would enable me to work at the preschool in the early part of the week. I felt that continuing my job was therapeutic for me, and it was something I didn't want to give up. But later, I began to feel as if I had really robbed my family by doing it that way. I lost weekends with them, and I lost mealtimes, which had always been one of the most important times for our family. It was normally a time to sit around talking and laughing together. But it got to the point where the smell of food would send me away from the table and back to the bathroom.

By my third round of chemotherapy, I had lost quite a bit of weight. My white blood count was going steadily down and my immune system was compromised. My level of nausea rendered me less and less functional, and the two other antinausea drugs I tried did absolutely nothing to help.

After the next round, something wonderful happened. A pediatric oncology nurse gave me a small bag of marijuana, and she told me it might help me. So I took it home and I tried it that night. After I took a few small hits, I immediately felt less nauseous. In a few minutes, I felt relief and I was able to fall asleep.

The next morning, I woke up feeling horrible as usual. It was normal on these mornings that I would have to make trip after trip to the bathroom. But after two or three hits of marijuana, there was a dramatic difference in the way I felt. The nausea usually lasted a few days unabated. But this time, I could cook for my family, and I was able to go back to work by Monday morning.

I decided to discuss my marijuana use with my oncologist, my surgeon, and my primary physician. They were all visibly relieved that I was getting some kind of relief from my nausea, and that I would be able to continue with my treatments.

For the remaining rounds of therapy, I continued to smoke marijuana in very small amounts, at the beginning of the day and at mealtimes. Usually, it enabled me to eat. I think it's what kept me hanging on. By the end of my treatment, my system had become more weakened. I developed sores in my mouth. I had double vision sometimes, and I began to experience a ringing in my ears. As I became more weak and debilitated, my nausea grew more intense. I don't think I would have been able to get to the end without marijuana.

By the end of my treatment, in 1990, my cancer was considered to be in remission. My prognosis was that if I were to remain in remission for seven years, I would probably remain cancer free. I feel very fortunate that, to this day, I have. Many of us who have breast cancer do not make it. In my cancer support group there were ten of us who were meeting in the beginning, and only five of us have survived.

I have to say that one of the most demoralizing points during my treatment was when I came up against the kind of prejudice that is part of drug education in this country. Our children get filled with it in their schools.

One day my ten-year-old son discovered some of the marijuana I had stashed in a small bag. He became angry at me, and he asked if it meant that the police were going to come take me away. Talk about sending the wrong message to our kids. I explained to my son that there was a great deal of difference between abusing marijuana and using it medically. I told him about some of the other legal and illegal drugs doctors can prescribe, and what they can do for people, when they're not abused.

After some time, both of my children came to understand. They had witnessed the benefit I received from this medicine. In all truth, the message that they got was that their mother was able to survive. Anything else they might be told in school, quite frankly, I think is sick and cruel.

When I saw how confused my kids were by the scare tactics at the center of most drug education, it led me to be more committed to letting people know the facts. I wanted to put more effort into supporting Proposition 215 in California. And I'm glad that I did. Marijuana has not only helped me, it's helped many other people to survive cancer and other life-threatening diseases.

I have an old school friend who has multiple sclerosis. She used to suffer with terrible muscle spasms, but she started smoking marijuana and it has made an incredible difference. She was someone who had never smoked marijuana in her life.

I'll never regret the decisions I have made, though there are those who'll say that they were wrong. I have survived a disease that takes the lives of thousands of women every year. Marijuana was the medicine that enabled me to do so.

Another patient, Michael Ferrucci of Livermore, California, discovered marijuana when he began chemotherapy for testicular cancer in 1992. Marijuana controlled his nausea and allowed him to conduct a normal, active life. However, he, too, was forced to overcome the conflict surrounding the use of an illegal medicine.

In 1992, I was diagnosed with testicular cancer. The cancer had metastasized to my lungs and caused lesion (tumors) in my chest. Within six months, I underwent four cycles of chemotherapy at Stanford Medical Center. I don't know how to describe the bouts of nausea I would get a few hours after each treatment. Anyone who has experienced it knows what it's like. You start to sweat, and you begin to feel an incredible anxiety. You know in just a few minutes you're going to begin vomiting, only you end up dry heaving, which is more painful because there's nothing left in your stomach.

I dreaded those few hours more than anything I can remember. I would end up on the floor by the toilet, or in the shower crying, with my family standing by. After each episode, I became more and more weak and dehydrated. I didn't know how long I could go on like that. It was the most painful experience of my life, but I had to bear it in order to continue chemotherapy.

For a while I used standard drugs like Compazine (Stemetil or Buccastem) and Zofran (ondansetron) to treat my nausea. The Zofran was somewhat effective but it cost $150 (about £105) per dose and it made me feel cloudy. In the hospital they had me on Marinol all of the time. I had to take it two hours before each chemotherapy treatment because it took nearly that long to work. It really wasn't very good medicine because the duration and the potency of its psychological effect made it almost nontherapeutic. There were times when it made me feel paranoid. Marinol simply never worked for me the way marijuana does when it first takes effect, so I couldn't use it to treat my bouts of nausea. When the Marinol did kick in, I felt nearly disabled, and this feeling lasted for hours, sometimes even into the next day.

I wanted to use marijuana in the hospital but couldn't. The doctors knew I was using it on my own, and there was a consensus among them that it worked, but they weren't allowed even to recommend it.

Before we began living with cancer, my wife and I had always been active people. We were enthusiastically involved in the lives of our three children. Even during my treatment, I wanted to continue living the way I always had. I still attended City Council meetings. I took my kids to school every day. I went to PTA meetings, and I eventually served as their Vice

President. But, more than ever, knowing I could survive chemotherapy, I felt like I wanted to make a difference in this world. I wanted to get out there and do something. I decided to run for Livermore City Council in 1995.

My use of medical marijuana helped me to keep my life. I could control my bouts of nausea with just a few puffs on a marijuana cigarette. Nothing worked faster or better. I thank God for it. It saved my life. But, soon, what became more of a problem for me than the chemotherapy was the stress – knowing that what I was doing to help myself would bring judgment or disapproval from my community. I realized this was only because they could not understand. But, when you are surviving chemotherapy, you're already undergoing a great deal of anxiety and stress, and you don't need any more. Marijuana is illegal, so it was stressful for me to use, no matter how effective it was.

I hope you can agree that it shouldn't be stressful for someone who is ill to use medicine that works. The social stigma around marijuana is cruel and unfair to those who need it for medicine. Because of this stigma, our medicine becomes public. If someone is injecting insulin for severe diabetes to maintain their health everyday, it's a private issue. I think marijuana should be private, too.

As you can see, many patients feel confused about why medical marijuana use has been legally prohibited, given that more is known about the safety of marijuana than most legally prescribed drugs. Patients who have lived with this confusion have come to feel, correctly, that their inability to use marijuana medicinally has everything to do with politics and little to do with science or medicine.

Interest in the medical usefulness of marijuana peaked following the first clinical tests at Harvard. As physicians and patients demanded more information, over 35 states passed legislation establishing medical marijuana research programmes. These programmes were later suppressed by federal drug regulations. In 1970, the American Congress passed the Controlled Substances Act, which classified marijuana as a Schedule I drug. That meant it was dangerous and had no known medical properties. Schedule I drugs cannot be used for any purpose without prior approval from both the Drug Enforcement Administration (DEA) and the Food and Drug Administration (FDA). This conflict with federal regulations effectively halted further scientific research under the state programmes.

Despite the legal restrictions, the medical use of marijuana in the US has increased over the last 20 years. This happened in part because the state-sponsored research programmes created a substantial body of evidence that marijuana worked in reducing nausea and vomiting, and stimulating appetite. In a study at Johns Hopkins University, smoked marijuana was found to increase the caloric intake of normal subjects by 40 per cent, resulting in significant increases in body weight (Foltin, 1986).

The political issues surrounding marijuana use have prevented cancer doctors from coming to a consensus regarding the use of marijuana to control nausea and vomiting from chemotherapy. Nonetheless, many patients, doctors and nurses commonly speak of the unwritten, unspoken acceptance of marijuana use by those receiving cancer chemotherapy. More and more patients are coming forward to question the legal status of medical marijuana. Many have testified that they first tried marijuana at the suggestion of doctors, nurses or other patients who knew that marijuana worked.

In the UK, studies are under way, but for the time being marijuana remains a Schedule I drug, and illegal both to possess or use. But doctors do continue to use Cesamet for cancer-treatment-related nausea and vomiting, and many patients (up to a quarter) claim that their doctors are aware of and either turn a blind eye to or outright approve of its use.

In 1990, Harvard researchers conducted a survey among a random sample of cancer doctors who were members of the American Society of Clinical Oncology. The researchers wanted to measure the attitudes and experiences of cancer specialists on the use of marijuana for nausea induced by chemotherapy. More than 70 per cent of the cancer doctors who responded reported that at least one of their patients had used marijuana to relieve nausea, and that they had directly observed or discussed such use with the patient. More surprising, 44 per cent of these doctors said that they had recommended the illegal use of marijuana to at least one of their patients (Doblin, 1991). The fact that so many doctors would illegally recommend marijuana to their patients points to a discrepancy between oncologists' experience with marijuana, and regulatory policies controlling it.

These statistics echo the feelings in the UK, where at least 25 per cent of doctors, claim one study, are prepared to look the other way and tolerate or even encourage the use of marijuana.

In 1985, the American Food and Drug Administration approved THC (Marinol), the main psychoactive ingredient in marijuana, for the treatment of nausea associated with cancer chemotherapy. A year later, oncologists were legally permitted to prescribe THC, which is marketed under the name Marinol. This drug is not licensed in the UK, although another cannabinoid, Nabilone, is. We pointed out in Chapter 3 that for a variety of reasons many patients don't like to take Marinol. As Jo Daly stated in her account above, Marinol failed to adequately alleviate her symptoms. In the same survey of members of the American Society of Clinical Oncology in

1990, cancer doctors were asked to compare the effectiveness of Marinol and smoked marijuana. Of the 277 oncologists who felt familiar enough with both drugs to respond, only 13 per cent thought Marinol worked better. In contrast, 44 per cent said they believed smoked marijuana to be better, and 43 per cent thought they were about equally effective (Doblin, 1991).

If you are a cancer patient who is considering using marijuana, it might help to know that many oncologists would support you. If your current oncologist refuses to discuss the option of marijuana with you, then talk to your GP about seeking other assistance. For more information on THC (Marinol), reread the section in Chapter 3 entitled, 'Synthetic THC (Marinol)'.

Chapter 5
AIDS and HIV

Acquired immunodeficiency syndrome (AIDS) refers to a specific group of diseases or conditions resulting from severe suppression of the immune system. The immune system is one of the body's defence mechanisms against infections and cancers. Scientists have identified the human immunodeficiency virus, or HIV, to be the infectious agent causing AIDS. HIV destroys the immune system by attacking a blood cell called a CD4 T-cell lymphocyte (or just T-cell). HIV in adults is spread by exposure to infected blood that may occur through sexual contact (homosexual or heterosexual), needle sticks (intravenous drug users or accidents among medical personnel) and, rarely, from transfused blood products. In the medical diagnosis and treatment of AIDS, the level of T-cells in the blood can indicate how far the disease has progressed.

In 1981, the first five cases of AIDS were reported in the United States. Shortly thereafter, the disease was categorized as an epidemic. By 1993, HIV infection was the most common cause of death among persons aged 25 to 44. According to the Centers for Disease Control and Prevention in America, there are approximately 650,000 to 900,000 HIV infected people living in the US, and nearly 220,000 people diagnosed with AIDS symptoms today. Tragically, over 320,000 Americans with AIDS have already died.

In the UK, the first official report of AIDS occurred in 1983, when three people died. By 1987, the World Health

Organization (WHO) reported that there were nearly 7500 known cases in Europe alone. Just three years later that number had jumped to over 41,500 with an estimated 500,000 patients with HIV in Europe.

In the UK, there was a total of 32,242 cases of HIV recorded between 1985 and 1996. Over the same period 15,565 patients were diagnosed with AIDS.

In total, 11,280 people have died from AIDS in the UK between the first recorded notification of the disease and March 1998.

The proportion of women with HIV rose from 13 to 21 per cent between 1993 and 1997.

By March 1998, a total of 626 children in the UK under 14 years of age were known to have been infected with HIV; 327 have been diagnosed with AIDS.

Like chemotherapy for cancer patients, the standard treatments for HIV infection are highly toxic. The drug conventionally used to treat HIV infection is zidovudine (AZT). This is an antiviral drug that slows the progression of the disease by attacking HIV. Unfortunately, AZT can have damaging effects on the digestive system and can cause the formation of kidney stones. It also causes significant nausea, so patients have difficulty withstanding treatment. The nausea also heightens the loss of appetite and weight that is associated with AIDS. This can lead to a condition known as AIDS wasting syndrome. Wasting syndrome is one of the leading causes of death from AIDS, as it leaves the body weak and susceptible to rare cancers and unusual infections.

In 1996, the Food and Drug Administration (FDA) approved the use of protease inhibitors that interfere with duplication of the HIV by blocking the activity of an enzyme called protease (Proteinase). They have made a sweeping change in AIDS therapy over the past two years. When taken in combination with conventional drugs like AZT and lamivudine (3TC), protease inhibitors can reduce HIV in the blood to very low levels, and slow the progression from HIV infection to the actual clinical symptoms of AIDS. This type of treatment is commonly referred to as triple therapy. This therapy is also available in the UK, and approved by the Medicines Control Board.

If you have HIV and have access to treatment with protease inhibitors, you should know that there are some drawbacks and concerns involved with their use. To begin with, these drugs are expensive. In the US, they can cost patients more than $15,000 (about £10,000) per year. As a result, they are out of reach for many people with HIV and AIDS. While this problem does not exist for individual patients in the UK, the treatment places a huge burden on the NHS and is used sparingly. Doctors have found that protease inhibitors do not work for all patients. In some, substantial levels of HIV remain in the blood following treatment. Those for whom triple therapy works can still experience problems when taking protease inhibitors in conjunction with other drugs, such as those commonly used to treat tuberculosis.

A concern for many who take protease inhibitors is that the side-effects can be more severe than those associated with AZT and 3TC alone. Like some cancer patients, many patients with AIDS find that the medicines they need to sustain their lives can produce side-effects so intolerable they become reluctant to maintain their treatment, or they fail to take treatment regularly. This can be dangerous because some research suggests that failure to maintain a regular medication schedule can lead to the development of strains of HIV that are no longer susceptible to drug treatment, a phenomenon called resistance. Not only would this pose a problem for the treatment of the individual patient, but it could also jeopardize the treatment of HIV infection generally if such resistant strains become widespread.

That patients with AIDS often comprise the majority of the members of cannabis (marijuana) buyers' clubs in many US cities indicates the failure of modern medicine to deal with the painful and undesirable side-effects of AIDS treatment. In the UK, cannabinoids are not yet licensed for the treatment of AIDS-related illnesses, but there is evidence that many sufferers do use cannabis therapeutically – with or without the approval of their doctors.

Service users at London Lighthouse, the charity for people with HIV and AIDS, are backing the movement to legalize cannabis for medicinal purposes, and have joined forces with ACT (Alliance 8 Cannabis Therapeutics). Cancer patients have long relied on marijuana to treat their nausea and weight loss and now, in growing numbers, people suffering from AIDS are turning to marijuana to treat the same symptoms. They are also using marijuana to treat their muscle spasms, chronic fatigue and pain. It is reasonable to conclude that with the rise in the epidemic over the last two decades, and with the increased toxicity of AIDS treatments, the number of people using marijuana to medicate themselves will continue to increase.

Steve Connell has been living with AIDS for the past nine years. Six years after Steve tested positive for HIV, his health deteriorated dramatically. Within weeks, he lost 40 pounds (17 kg, or nearly 3 stones) and tired so easily, he could no longer work. He grew severely depressed and despondent and he was ready to give up on life. Fortunately, recently available medications helped turn Steve's condition around. In the following account, he relates how he would not have been able to tolerate these new medications without the aid of marijuana:

> I learned I was HIV-positive in 1988, after suffering for some time with chronic diarrhea. I was at work when I found out. I felt so devastated, my head began spinning. I had to leave

immediately. From work, I went straight over to my girlfriend's house to break it off with her because I was afraid of the danger I was putting her in. A part of me really wanted her to get as far away from me as she could. But when I told her the news, and what I thought we should do, she said she wanted to face the situation together. She even suggested that we get married.

We married within the next six months and she was tested for HIV regularly. Luckily, every test came out negative. I thank God each day that she stood by me, and that she did not also contract this nightmare of a disease. For the first five or six years, I couldn't acknowledge my sickness to anyone other than my wife. Though it's not as bad today, there is a stigma around this disease. The first thing people want to know when they find out you have it, is what you could have done to get it. Because of that stigma, and because I didn't want it to change my life, I kept my sickness to myself.

I began having real problems in 1994. I had been the sports and entertainments writer for the old *Sacramento Union*, until the entire paper went belly up. Then I took a job as a page designer at the Alameda Newspaper Group. I had to commute 92 miles (147 km) to and from work every day, and I think it took a big toll on my health. I was taking AZT at the time, but it didn't seem to be helping me. There were times when I just couldn't take the pills because I was feeling too nauseous. I wasn't even eating food because I couldn't swallow anything without vomiting. Living like this, day after day, my body became run-down and weak.

That's when everything began to crumble. I tried to keep going. But after a few weeks, I just couldn't work anymore and I had to quit my job. It was as if my body was giving up on me. I was in intense pain, and I felt constantly nauseous. On top of that, I was frightened by what was happening to my life and I knew I could no longer keep my condition to myself.

I was going to have to tell my children that I had AIDS. This disease had taken over my life, and it was going to take over part of theirs, as well. I didn't want them finding out from anyone else. When I told them, they were quite young, and it took a few years for them to really understand. My daughter, who was 15 years old, just broke down in tears. My son took the news quietly. Years later, he told me he'd always wished I hadn't told him as early as I did. I know it deeply changed both of them.

Within eight months, beginning in 1995, I was hospitalized three times for pneumonia and sinus infection. I'd been feeling pain and congestion in my chest, and then I began having trouble breathing. I was still taking AZT and they put me on antibiotics and prednisone for the pneumonia. It was so difficult for me to swallow the pills. Almost immediately after taking them, a violent nausea would set in. I couldn't eat or hold down any food. After a few weeks of this, my weight dropped down from 150 pounds (67 kg) to 115 (51 kg). Soon I became seriously depressed, so they added an antidepressant to my list of pills. At this point, I had pretty much given up and resigned myself to death.

I did what I could during that time to get relief. That's when I realized, almost coincidentally, that marijuana alleviated my nausea. Soon, I began smoking it regularly. When I took a few hits of marijuana, I felt better within five to fifteen minutes. Usually the better the quality of marijuana, the better it worked. It also gave me back my appetite. In a short time, I gained back almost all my weight, and I began feeling much healthier.

Just as importantly, my marijuana use would help me deal with the new drugs I'd soon be taking. They began combining AZT and another antiviral drug, called 3TC (Lamivudine, not available in the UK), with a protease inhibitor called Crixivan (indinavir sulphate). I did notice a gradual improvement in my health, and my T-cell count started coming up. But the nausea I experienced was worse than anything I had felt with AZT alone. It was indescribable. It didn't seem like I have many choices though. I knew I needed these medicines to stay alive, even though the nausea they caused me was unbearable. So I kept taking them, along with marijuana to control the nausea.

I have to tell you that I sincerely doubt I could have continued the treatment without marijuana. This is very important because, while there is no cure for AIDS, I believe these medications have actually reversed my disease and saved my life. What marijuana did, aside from making me feel better, was make these drugs tolerable for me.

Because marijuana was illegal, I tried getting Marinol. But my doctor wouldn't prescribe it to me. I then tried talking to him about my marijuana use, and he made it clear that he wished to remain neutral. He did not agree with my marijuana use, but he could not disagree with it either. So I continued to smoke marijuana without the advice or consent of my doctor.

Right now, my weight is up to 148 pounds (65 kg). I take 16 pills a day, and I smoke marijuana before each meal to quell the nausea and stimulate my appetite. About one half-hour before I want to eat, I take three or four puffs. Usually, in about 20 minutes, I get the munchies and then I want to eat. It's still a struggle sometimes, but I'm healthier, stronger, and I enjoy living.

The difference marijuana has helped to make is that with it I have quality of life again, and hope, whereas before I did not. When I was real sick, I didn't think I would ever live to be 40. Now I plan on being around for my children when I'm 50, maybe older. I feel optimistic that they will find better and more lasting treatments for AIDS. It seems they're making new breakthroughs all the time.

I'll admit that because I've had respiratory problems, I have been concerned about smoking marijuana. I've even quit smoking tobacco cigarettes recently. Some time ago, I tried eating cannabis (marijuana) in food instead. But it was too difficult to do when I felt so nauseous. Since then, my health has improved because I've been able to take my pills, and I eat regularly. I feel I can experiment again with marijuana in foods until I figure out what will work for me.

Yes, marijuana does work. I am living proof, and I know hundreds of other people who are, too. We are aware that there may be detrimental effects of smoking, but taking that risk is a better option than the alternative. I don't want to be 115 pounds (51 kg) again and waiting for my death. I'm willing to put up with the legal hassle and the possible risks for the quality of life I get in return. And I'm grateful for every day that I have. It's unfortunate that it takes something like this to help you appreciate the little things, and to know just how precious your life really is. I don't understand how anyone could want to take that away from me.

At one point during his battle with AIDS, Greg Scott's doctor advised him that marijuana had become a necessary part of his treatment. Greg was losing too much weight due to wasting syndrome and a parasite in the intestine. At that point, marijuana was the only thing able to help Greg maintain his weight.

I learned about the medicinal potential of marijuana before I ever needed it. I watched my friend with AIDS suffering from nausea and wasting syndrome until he died in 1988. When Ray found out he had AIDS, it was the height of the Reagan–Bush 'Just Say No', era, and he had decided he was going to clean up his life. First, he stopped drinking and smoking, which only seemed to benefit his health. But in order to do this, he followed a 12-step program that required him to quit smoking marijuana, as well. This was the last thing Ray wanted to give up. Once he did, his daily struggle with severe nausea began. He soon had trouble taking his medication. He couldn't eat anything and he began losing weight quite dramatically.

In spite of the opinions of those around him who were watching him waste away so badly, Ray never went back to using marijuana. Within a year, I saw him grow increasingly more sick until, one day, he was gone. I stored it all away in my memory.

I was diagnosed HIV positive just before Ray, but my condition was far less progressed than his. The US Navy tested me in 1987, as part of a command screening. I found out later that they had launched an investigation into my sexuality before even telling me I was HIV positive.

After I was kicked out of the Navy, I went back home to Washington, DC, where I worked for a little while. I needed to wrestle with the information I had just learned, and figure out how I was going to live the rest of my life. During that time, I came across a group that was working to sign people on to the government's 'Compassionate Use' program. I had known the federal government was cultivating marijuana since I was a kid growing up in Oxford, Mississippi. We used to build forts along the edge of the woods, near the government pot farm that was located near the University. Given the new circumstances of my life, the idea of getting safe and legal marijuana from the government was very attractive to me. But the program was canceled before I could even apply.

I began using marijuana regularly when I was taking AZT. It relieved my nausea and calmed my stomach after taking a handful of pills every morning. It also gave me a healthy appetite. I tried other appetite enhancers but they were too difficult to take. I tried Marinol, too, but aside from being difficult to swallow, it was too high a dosage for me. It might have been enjoyable for someone interested in recreational use, but it was not amusing to me when I was trying just to live. Marinol also cost me about $600 (about £420) a month and, although the state paid for most of it through Medicaid, I was angry that the government could force people to use such an ineffective and costly substance. Marijuana was so much less expensive and it really worked.

Marijuana also had the added effect of relieving my pain, but I didn't realize this until a little later. One of the most dramatic experiences I've ever had using marijuana has been to feel the way it eases the pain in my hands and feet from neuropathy. It worked differently than the painkillers my doctor was giving me. These drugs seemed to cover up the pain rather than relieve it.

Another consequence of wasting syndrome is that your body becomes vulnerable to opportunistic infections, of which I had several. One of these was actually bringing about my death. I had a gastrointestinal parasite called microsporidia. This was something they discovered was causing severe wasting in many patients with AIDS. It was causing me to starve to death. I went from 160 to 120 pounds (71 to 53 kg) in weight. I had no T-cells and an alarmingly high viral load.

At that point my doctor and I began talking about my need just to stay alive. We had to do something to improve my immune system overall, or find something that would attack this microscopic parasite directly. During that time, my doctor advised me that marijuana was crucial to my health because every pound I lost seemed to equal a lost day of my life. Marijuana was the only thing helping me to maintain any weight and he knew this. He had several other patients who were using it, too. I asked him to put his knowledge of my need for marijuana in writing, in case I would ever have any legal problems.

There were two things that eventually caused my health to make a complete turn around. In 1995, I got access to a highly controlled substance called thalidomide. This was the drug that could fight my parasite. Shortly after that, they made protease inhibitors available. I began taking both the thalidomide and the protease inhibitor, and within six weeks they could no longer find the parasite in me. Both of these drugs dramatically changed my condition, but I believe that if I had not used marijuana, I would have died before they ever came along.

Marijuana enabled me to continue the treatments that made me well. Now my T-cell count is up to about 300, and my viral load is almost immeasurable. It's taken a lot for me to be here still. For anyone who is in my place, every life-saving choice is precious. That's why people should have a right to know the truth about marijuana. I don't think marijuana use should be taken lightly, but I do think it should be taken seriously for its medicinal value.

Regarding the effects that marijuana is said to have on the immune system, I have a few big problems with the claims I've heard. The first is that such contradictory conclusions have been drawn. There hasn't been enough research to determine the truth. But all of that aside, when I was in the grip of AIDS, with no T-cells in my blood, marijuana provided me a great deal of comfort.

Even if I was not recovering, the relief would have been worth any bad effect the marijuana might have had. I could keep down food, and I could stop the aching. Also, I'm convinced that one of the worst things for my immune system was the stress my sickness caused me. Marijuana reduced my stress and it calmed my soul. It made me not worry so much

> about the difficult regimen of pills I had to take, or how I was going to get to the grocery store because I didn't think I'd be able to walk. Marijuana allowed me to accept the possibility that I might die, and yet, I believe, because I smoked marijuana, I lived.

Thousands of people living with AIDS are using marijuana daily because it works. Yet, the drug bureaucracy has kept a virtual stranglehold on all research into its safety and effectiveness. At the University of California in San Francisco, AIDS researcher, Dr Donald Abrams, wanted to do a study to compare the effectiveness of Marinol versus smoked marijuana. The Food and Drug Administration (FDA) granted approval to launch the study. However, under federal law, all marijuana used in research must come from the federal marijuana farm in Mississippi that is under the control of the National Institute on Drug Abuse (NIDA). NIDA denied Dr Abrams access to the marijuana he needed for his FDA-approved research project.

More recently, following the passage of Proposition 215 in California, and the resulting increased pressure on the US government to allow marijuana research, Abrams finally got the green light and is proceeding with a scaled-down version of his original research proposal. The political pressure created by Proposition 215, along with public opinion polling that shows a majority of Americans to be sympathetic to medical marijuana use, is slowly forcing US officials to moderate their long-held opposition to marijuana research. In the UK, public opinion and the pressure of lobby groups have forced the government to extend cannabis research licences, but at present they have only sanctioned the study of pain control and multiple sclerosis treatment. We believe it is criminal for the government to obstruct clinical research when tens of thousands of people are currently using marijuana for its medicinal benefits. Worse, tens of thousands more might be able to use marijuana as medicine if governments accepted its obvious benefits and ended the criminal sanctions imposed on those patients who do.

Until now, barring scientific inquiry into the medicinal uses of marijuana has effectively denied patients knowledge that may be useful to them. Instead, they were left with contradictory claims about its safety and effectiveness. For example, from the beginning of the epidemic, opponents of the medicinal use of marijuana have argued that it is particularly harmful to people with AIDS because of adverse effects on the immune system. This followed unconfirmed reports in the early 1970s that marijuana weakened the body's response to disease.

Following these reports, several researchers tried to find supporting evidence. In one such study, Gabriel Nahas tested the effect of marijuana on the body's immune function, using T-cells extracted from the blood of both marijuana users and nonusers. Nahas claimed to find evidence that marijuana weakened the immune system, making the body more susceptible to disease (Zimmer and Morgan, 1997; 107–108). However, other researchers could not duplicate Dr Nahas's results. More recently, a National Institutes of Health scientific panel concluded that while the unique compounds found in marijuana called cannabinoids do suppress some immune responses, they also tend to enhance others. In particular, there has been no evidence that cannabinoids actually harm or reduce the number of T-cells in people infected with HIV.

Despite the questions raised about his research results, Nahas's conclusion is still promoted by those government officials and private groups who are opposed to marijuana use. Nonetheless, in 1992, the Food and Drug Administration officially approved the use of synthetic THC (Marinol) in the treatment of AIDS wasting syndrome. This contradictory action obviously calls into question any government or private claims about marijuana suppressing the immune system. In the UK, no cannabinoid is licensed for the treatment of AIDS or related illnesses.

Marinol won FDA approval because orally administered THC has relieved nausea and increased appetite in clinical studies with AIDS patients. In a 1991 study, Marinol relieved nausea and produced weight gain in 70 per cent of participating patients (Grinspoon, 1997; 102). Following the study, about one-fifth of the patients who benefited from Marinol discontinued their use of it because of unwanted side-effects. Like many cancer patients, people with AIDS have expressed a preference for smoked marijuana over Marinol because it provides results with smaller doses and fewer undesirable side-effects. Reread the section on Marinol in Chapter 3 for more information.

The risk of potential respiratory and lung infection from smoking marijuana is a real concern for people with AIDS, who are thought to be more susceptible because of their weakened immune systems. The results of a study at Johns Hopkins University in the US showed that patients with AIDS who smoked illicit drugs, including marijuana and cocaine, were twice as likely to contract pneumocystis carinii pneumonia (PCP) than those who did not smoke marijuana (Rosenthal, 1997; 37). Though it should be mentioned that most of the subjects in the study also smoked tobacco cigarettes, people with AIDS should be cautious about smoking marijuana. Long-term heavy use may lower resistance to respiratory infections.

Another risk associated with marijuana use results from the possibility that the marijuana may be contaminated with bacteria or fungal spores. This can be particularly dangerous for patients with AIDS. Some patients minimize this risk by cultivating their own marijuana. Others are careful to obtain their marijuana only from trusted sources. In Chapter 20, we'll describe some ways to sterilize marijuana in order to avoid the risk from contamination.

Some patients try to reduce the risk of using contaminated marijuana by alternately smoking marijuana and cooking it in food. They rely on smoked marijuana when the symptoms of nausea are so severe they are incapable of ingesting it. At other times, they bake it into brownies or other food. In this way, when necessary, they can get the immediate and effective relief that smoking provides, but when the need is less pressing, they can minimize the risk of smoking potentially contaminated marijuana.

Marijuana has helped many patients prolong their lives by enabling them to cope with some of the difficult symptoms and treatments associated with AIDS, and by helping them to maintain their body weight. Though rigorous scientifically controlled research is lacking, patients with AIDS are using marijuana in growing numbers because they feel nothing works better. Among the most vocal groups demanding the right to use medical marijuana are the many organizations of AIDS patients and AIDS caregivers. If you are HIV positive or living with AIDS, and you are considering using marijuana, you may want to seek information and advice from such groups.

Chapter 6
Glaucoma

Glaucoma is a disease that occurs when the drainage system in the eye becomes blocked, thus preventing the nourishing fluid that is constantly produced inside the eyeball from flowing out. As excessive amounts of this fluid build up inside the eyeball, there is an increase in pressure. This is called intra-ocular pressure because it is the pressure inside the eye. In glaucoma, intra-ocular pressure rises to abnormally high levels. When intra-ocular pressure gets too high, or remains at high levels for too long, it can cause permanent damage to the retina and the optic nerve. Because the optic nerve carries all visual information from the retina to the brain, this can often result in impairment or even total loss of vision. In fact, glaucoma is the leading cause of blindness in America today, affecting approximately two million people. In the UK, some form of glaucoma affects about two in 100 people over the age of 40, and is responsible for about 15 per cent of blindness in adults.

There are two main types of glaucoma. Chronic, or open-angle, glaucoma is the most common type, accounting for at least 90 per cent of all cases. Chronic glaucoma progresses slowly over a long period of time. Excess fluid builds up in the eye, gradually raising the level of intra-ocular pressure. Usually, there are no noticeable symptoms. This puts the patient's vision at risk because the increased pressure is likely to go untreated. Without treatment, it is common for people who have chronic glaucoma to have their vision clouded by halos and blind spots. The longer they go without treatment, the more likely they are to lose their peripheral, and then their central or primary, vision.

If you have been diagnosed with chronic glaucoma, you will need constant medical treatment to prevent your intra-ocular pressure from reaching dangerously high levels. Most doctors will prescribe pills or eyedrops to reduce your intra-ocular pressure. If this treatment proves inadequate, you may be encouraged to undergo surgery. It is important that you are informed about all available options so you can choose the treatment best for you. Your vision may be at stake. Marijuana is another option that many people with chronic glaucoma have chosen.

Acute, or closed-angle, glaucoma is less common and usually more severe than chronic glaucoma. People with acute glaucoma experience extreme eye pain, headaches, nausea and blurred vision. Surgical treatment is more commonly required to preserve eyesight. Marijuana is not considered to be as useful in treating this type of glaucoma because its progression is much more rapid and difficult to control. Nevertheless, some people with acute glaucoma find marijuana helpful in treating the pain and nausea they suffer.

In the past, many of the drugs routinely prescribed for glaucoma were inadequate or caused serious side-effects in many patients. Eyedrops that were promoted as effective glaucoma medication often failed to control intra-ocular pressure and sometimes increased the risk of hypertension, respiratory problems, reduced heart rate, and even heart failure. Oral medications often caused nausea, vomiting, loss of appetite, headaches, kidney stones and blood disorders. Surgical procedures sometimes failed and needed to be repeated. They also involved some risk of serious complications, such as permanent damage to the eye and loss of vision.

New prescription drugs have been developed, among them timolol (Timoptol) and latanoprost (Xalatan), which are claimed to be highly effective and have few side-effects. Unfortunately, some patients are finding that these drugs do have side-effects, or that they do not sufficiently reduce intra-ocular pressure. While Timoptol helps to reduce intra-ocular pressure in most cases, it can cause asthma and can affect heart rate and heart muscle function. This is an even more serious concern for patients over the age of 35, which includes most glaucoma victims. Xalatan can change the colour of the eyes. Some patients who take these medications must still undergo numerous surgical procedures. Many doctors agree that the difficulties with these treatments probably result from the fact that patients vary both in their severity of intra-ocular pressure and their response to medication.

If you have glaucoma, you may experience similar difficulty in your treatment. You are not alone. There are many people suffering from glaucoma who were frustrated with their treatment options and chose to use marijuana as their medicine. They believe marijuana has helped them to maintain a low level of intra-ocular pressure and prevent further damage to their optic nerves. For some, marijuana has eliminated the appearance of halos and blind spots that impaired their vision. For others, marijuana relieved the pain that resulted from their glaucoma. Some patients have chosen marijuana simply because it is not painful or difficult to administer.

Bill Barrett is a glaucoma patient who chose to use marijuana for all of these reasons. He had witnessed his mother's lifelong struggle with glaucoma and her frustration with the array of failed glaucoma treatments she received. Bill faced the same options when he was diagnosed with glaucoma. Then he discovered that the marijuana he was using to cope with multiple sclerosis also provided an effective option for treating his glaucoma.

I found out that I had chronic, or open-angle, glaucoma when I was 32 years old, but it wasn't a surprise to me. My mother had glaucoma for which she'd been treated nearly all of her life, until she died at the age of 60. I always wondered if her death was somehow related to the medications she took over the years. The various types of eyedrops that were supposed to help control the pressure in her eyes were known to cause slowed heart rate, even heart failure. She never lost her sight, but she suffered four heart attacks before she eventually died of cardiac arrest.

Because glaucoma can be hereditary, I was routinely checked for it when I was growing up. As an adult, I had regular checkups and was considered borderline, until it showed up when I was 32. My doctors immediately started me on eyedrops, which they changed several times throughout my treatment. I remember my mother used to complain because she had to take the drops two times a day and she hated it. She said they burned her eyes.

I knew these drugs had serious side-effects and, because of what had happened to my mother, I was concerned about what I was taking. So they put me on Betoptic and assured me that it had no side-effects. Shortly after I began taking the Betoptic, the pressure in my eye elevated way up to somewhere in the 30s. Then they gave me an ointment that had to be applied onto my eyelids every evening. This medicine took effect almost immediately, but it blurred my vision to the point of total blindness, which lasted for several hours.

Now, I know they say that there are newer, more potent drugs that have no side-effects. But I have not found this to be true. I've tried Timoptol, and it did work to reduce my pressure. But it's extremely expensive and may cause cardiac arrest. The last prescription they gave me was something called Trusopt (dorzolamide), but it did nothing to lower the level of my pressure.

In spite of all the medications they were giving me, my pressure continued to increase until, a little more than eight years ago, my doctor was afraid I was going to go blind. She told me that I needed surgery. Luckily, I wouldn't agree to it even though it seemed there was nothing else I could do.

By that time, I had begun to use high grade marijuana more regularly to treat my multiple sclerosis. It wasn't very long before I noticed it was also helping me with my glaucoma. I remember the first time I went in for an examination after smoking marijuana. My doctor thought a miracle had happened. My pressure had gone down from the 30s to 13 or 14 since the last time I'd seen her. When I told her I was using marijuana, she was so amazed she began working with me to monitor the effects it was having on my pressure. There were times when I went in after periods of not having any marijuana, or using a very low grade type because it was all I could get. At those times, my pressure had shot up significantly.

After nearly ten years of working like this with my doctor, I don't understand why my experience doesn't count as evidence of marijuana's usefulness. If marijuana hadn't worked, I know my doctor wouldn't have accepted my use. But she did. Eventually, she gave me a written letter stating that she'd been following my battle with glaucoma, and that she'd seen it help me when nothing else could. She even stated that she would give me a prescription if it were legal.

I am now 52 years old, and I've used marijuana for the last ten years to treat my glaucoma. I smoke one joint every four or five hours, a little at a time. It continues to work the same each time for my pressure, but I don't get high from it anymore. It just relaxes me. I smoke because when I don't smoke the pressure in my eyes gets too high and I begin to see halos.

There are many things I don't like about smoking. I don't like the smell, and I don't like the fact that it's illegal. This makes things more difficult for a lot of people who are suffering. I've talked to other glaucoma patients who were losing their eyesight but wouldn't take marijuana because they were afraid of the law. I think marijuana may be a miracle drug, and it may be that people don't want to legalize it for that reason.

I've seen people helped by marijuana for many different things. Look at me. I've been able to stop the progression of both my diseases. The bottom line is that marijuana isn't painful to take, it doesn't cause any life-threatening side-effects, and it doesn't make me go blind. Instead, marijuana has helped me keep my vision. I'm grateful every day for that.

Jacqueline Mahone is a 41-year-old woman who was born with congenital glaucoma. This is a rare form of glaucoma that develops before birth and may be hereditary. In Jacqueline's case, it appears to have skipped several generations from a distant aunt and affected her. She was the only one of six children in her family born with it. In the following account, Jacqueline tells about a childhood of failed medical treatments and surgical procedures and how she discovered the benefit that came from the medicinal use of marijuana.

I had my first surgery when I was three years old. The doctors told my mother when I was born that I would eventually go blind. They said that with surgery they would only be able to relieve some of the pressure that was destroying my vision. She agreed to let them perform the surgery anyway because she wanted to preserve what little sight I did have for as long as possible.

I've heard of rare cases where people with glaucoma have had so much pressure build up, their eyeball couldn't take it anymore and it burst. That didn't happen to me, but my doctors were afraid of what would happen at the rate my pressure was increasing. So they performed surgery on me about every six months until I was six years old.

As a child, I went through a period of several years when my condition was livable without surgery. During that time, living with glaucoma made me appreciate what I could see – light, shadows, and little bits of color. My mother always made sure I had the chance to experience these things when I could. She began to encourage my independence, to prepare me to live without my eyesight. She even had a woman from the church come to my home to teach me how to read Braille.

When I was 15, we were told I had to be seen by an ophthalmologist in order to receive government aid for the blind. I had already been, for some time, feeling pain again in my eyes. I was so afraid of going to the doctor to be examined and subjected to another treatment. After my first exam, the doctor told me what I'd been afraid of hearing. He said that I had developed polyps in my eyes, and they would probably get worse without another surgery. But I refused to have surgery and, soon, all I could see were large objects and a little bit of color.

My doctor began treating me with eyedrops, but they weren't working. All the surgical procedures I'd had as a child made it very difficult for me to put anything into my eyes. I always disliked having to hold my eyes open during examinations. I told my doctor that I wouldn't use the drops, but I couldn't bear to have another surgery. It was then that he told me about marijuana. My doctor said that marijuana had medical properties that might help my condition. He knew other patients who were helped by it. He'd also heard that tests were underway to develop new eyedrops, made with one of the active ingredients in marijuana, called THC. He said he was hoping something like this would become available to me.

None of this meant very much to me at the time. I was leery about the whole idea of using marijuana for medicine, and I was not at all interested in trying any new type of eyedrops. Besides, I had never even tried using marijuana recreationally, as I had been brought up to avoid all drugs.

In high school, I was very socially active and popular with most of my peers. I was involved in all the student politics and had been elected vice president of the student body. Through my activities, I developed acquaintances with many different types of people. One day, in my sophomore year, some kids I knew had brought a marijuana joint to school, and they invited me to go up onto the roof and smoke it with them. At first, I didn't feel any different. But when I got down off the roof to go to history class, I started feeling rather clumsy and giddy. That was the first time I ever tried using marijuana, and I always remember it as a pleasant experience.

Soon, I entered a period of my life that was a minor divergence from where I had come. I embarked on the type of youthful experimentation that I think most people associate with that time in their lives. Nevertheless, I managed to stay on the honor roll at school, and I continued my participation in all the healthy social activities around me.

By the age of 17, I'd grown pretty independent and had a strong desire to move out on my own. My mother was concerned but supportive, so she allowed me to move into a residential skill center for the blind. There I was given mobility instruction and taught different skills that would enable me to be more effective with my diminishing sight.

About a year after I moved into the center, I began having severe pain in my left eye, so I went back to see my doctor. He discovered that I had developed more polyps, and the condition of my left eye was deteriorating. My cornea was clouded, and I had almost no vision left. When I was in the hospital they gave me codeine and Demerol (meriperidine, or pethidine) for the pain, but these drugs did nothing to ease my pressure. When they wore off, the pain was still there. Eventually, it got so unbearable that I agreed to undergo another surgical procedure. This time, they froze the optic nerve in both my eyes so that I wouldn't feel the pain anymore.

Eventually, the nerves woke up and the pain came back. It was then, in my desperation, that I discovered that what had begun as occasional recreational marijuana use could actually help me cope. Marijuana was the only thing that gave me relief. After all the treatments I had been given, and the numerous surgical procedures I'd had since I was three years old, the pressure in my eyes had continued to cause irreversible damage. I was going to lose my vision. The only thing I could do now was deal with the pain. I was 25 years old, and I decided that I would never undergo another surgery. I would take no more of the medicines they prescribed. Marijuana was the only medicine I would use.

I thought my doctors should know about it, so I made them fully aware that I was using marijuana. Sure I had skeptics. But I also met many doctors and patients who shared experiences similar to mine. The doctor that I'd had since I was 15 told me he would even get marijuana for me if he could. And why couldn't he?

I'll never forget how I felt when I found out, in 1976, that there were people who were getting marijuana for medical use from the government. I wasn't upset because these people were able to get relief. I was upset because our government was acknowledging the medicinal value of marijuana, yet denying it to me and to many other people like me. I was forced to go out and obtain it illegally, in environments that were often alien and uncomfortable for me.

I am now 41 years old and I still use marijuana. People ask me why I choose to use it when there are other medicines available, and I have to tell them how I came to this choice. In my experience, marijuana worked better than anything else. And it still works. It relieves my pressure without the side-effects that legal medicines have. With marijuana, I feel the psychoactive effects, but they're not unpleasant and I know when to stop. Like any other drug, it changes the way I feel a little, but I'd rather have the feeling I get from marijuana than the pain any day.

University of California researchers discovered that marijuana could be useful for treating glaucoma in the early 1970s, after carrying out a study for the Los Angeles Police Department. The purpose of the experiment was to confirm the belief that the use of marijuana resulted in dilated pupils. Law enforcement officers commonly made this assumption in determining whether or not a suspected citizen was under the influence of marijuana. Each subject in the experiment was given federally grown marijuana and photographed while smoking. After smoking, they received ophthalmologic examinations. The photographs showed that rather than dilating, the subjects' pupils had constricted. The researchers also found that marijuana had reduced intra-ocular pressure and the production of tears (Grinspoon, 1997; 46–47).

A number of studies followed, confirming that marijuana effectively reduced intra-ocular pressure in glaucoma patients. On average, smoked marijuana was found to reduce pressure by about 30 per cent for a period of four to five hours. Intra-ocular pressure began to decrease within 30 minutes of inhalation, with the maximum decrease being reached in 60 to 90 minutes. There was no evidence that the effects were dependent on the dose, or that subjects developed any tolerance with continued use. In a New York study done in 1976, 29 subjects who smoked marijuana cigarettes for 94 days showed a reduction in intra-ocular pressure each time that they used marijuana (Green, 1983). These findings led to the belief that marijuana could be used in the long-term treatment of glaucoma because its effectiveness did not decrease over time.

Unfortunately, because of the politics that surround the use of marijuana, there have been no further studies to fully explore just how marijuana works to reduce intra-ocular pressure. The current understanding is that THC constricts the capillaries in the eye, decreasing the rate of fluid secretion. This can explain why people who use marijuana often report a reduction in tears and a drying of the eyes. THC is also thought to expand the blood vessels in the mucous membranes that facilitate the drainage of fluid from the eye. This may explain why marijuana smokers often appear to have bloodshot eyes.

Orally administered THC (Marinol) is legal, but cannot be prescribed for glaucoma. In any case, many patients believe it is not as effective as marijuana. Many glaucoma patients have claimed that Marinol simply does not work for them. In the same 1976 study done in New York, oral THC capsules were found to be effective only in very high doses. Using these high doses of synthetic oral THC, patients felt incapacitated and experienced unpleasant psychological effects. Tests using such high doses were eventually discontinued. Reread the section on Marinol in Chapter 3 for more information.

By the late 1970s, there was interest in developing a THC solution that could be administered in drops to the surface of the eye. The idea was favoured by ophthalmologists because a patient could apply THC without smoking it or experiencing any psychological effects. Unfortunately, no topical solution is yet available that would allow proper penetration and absorption of THC into the eye.

Smoking is not the only method of using marijuana to treat glaucoma. Many patients ingest marijuana in brownies or in other foods. Some people mix it in teas or tinctures. However you decide to use marijuana to treat your glaucoma, it is important that you consider the possible risks involved, and that you make the decision that is best for your glaucoma, as well as your overall health.

While medical research and patient experience point to the usefulness of marijuana in reducing intra-ocular pressure, it is still not officially accepted as a viable long-term treatment for glaucoma. Ophthalmologists remain concerned about the effects of long-term smoking on their patient's health. Glaucoma generally affects people above the age of 35, who are likely to be more vulnerable to respiratory problems caused by prolonged smoking. Even so, a panel of the National Institutes of Health recently suggested that further studies on marijuana would be useful in treating the many patients who fail to respond to standard therapies.

In a telling statement, however, the American Academy of Ophthalmology states on its web page that they are opposed to the use of marijuana in the treatment of glaucoma. In justifying their conclusion, they cited the unpleasant side-effects of smoking marijuana. The first such side-effect listed is 'euphoria'. A leading medical dictionary defines euphoria as 'bodily comfort or well-being' (*Dorland's*, 26th Edition; 471). How ironic that a drug which has proven to be so beneficial is passed over by doctors because it makes patients feel better.

Chapter 7
Multiple Sclerosis

An autoimmune disorder occurs when the body's immune system attacks its own tissues or cells. It is not known what causes this reaction, but it is thought that some cases are triggered by viral or bacterial infection. Multiple sclerosis, or MS, is an autoimmune disorder involving myelin, the protective covering around nerve fibres in the brain and spinal cord (or central nervous system). In particular, multiple sclerosis develops when the immune system mistakenly treats myelin as a foreign substance. White blood cells then attack and destroy patches of myelin, interrupting critical nerve impulses to and from the brain. The name multiple sclerosis refers to the patches of hardened scar tissue, or sclerosis, which form where myelin has been destroyed.

According to the National Multiple Sclerosis Society in the US, an estimated one-third of a million Americans live with MS and nearly 200 new cases are diagnosed each week. Across the world there are more than 2.5 million sufferers, about 85,600 of them in the UK. People with MS suffer a variety of symptoms due to problems with their central nervous system. These problems include blurred vision, slurred speech, loss of bladder and bowel control, problems with sexual function, generalized weakness and severe depression. Among the more debilitating symptoms are numbness, loss of coordination or balance, painful muscle spasm and tremors, and loss of movement control or paralysis. The particular symptoms that each MS patient endures relate to the location of the nerve damage and can occur nearly anywhere in the body.

MS affects individuals very differently. It is without consistent pattern, and can resemble other disorders of the central nervous system. There are, however, three general patterns of the MS disease, relapsing-remitting, secondary-progressive and chronic-progressive.

Relapsing-remitting MS is probably the most common pattern. It is characterized by unpredictable attacks or relapses, followed by periods of quiescence or remission. In remission, a patient's health may return to its original state for up to several years. Secondary-progressive MS is much like relapsing-remitting, except the patient's overall condition usually deteriorates further with each attack. Physical, mental or emotional stress may trigger a relapse. Chronic-progressive MS is the most severe pattern, in which the patient's condition steadily worsens without attacks or remissions, and results in partial or total disability. Finally, there is a fourth, benign, category for which most victims are never even diagnosed, as they will experience only minor symptoms once or twice in their lifetime.

Sadly, there is no known cure for multiple sclerosis. Patients are treated medically for their symptoms. Prednisone is a cortisone type of steroid hormone, and adrenocorticotropic hormone (ACTH) is a hormone that stimulates the body to produce its own cortisone. Thus, ACTH acts like cortisone when administered to treat MS. These powerful hormones are used to shut down the immune system during acute attacks. Unfortunately, these agents are often ineffective and may cause significant problems. Common side-effects include nausea and vomiting, mood swings, depression, sleeplessness, fluid retention with bloating and drastic weight gain. Long-term cortisone can also cause diabetes, cataracts, stomach problems, abnormal blood potassium levels, immune system breakdown, thinning of the bones (osteoporosis), redistribution of body fat which may change facial appearance, muscle atrophy and countless other problems. Additional medications with their own unique side-effects are often used to treat the complications of long-term cortisone use.

Over the past few years, nonsteroid drugs, such as Avonex (interferon beta IA), Betaferon (Betaseron or interferon beta IB) and Copolymer-1 (glatiramer acetate), have become increasingly popular in the treatment of multiple sclerosis. However, because they are fairly new, much about their activities in the body remains unknown.

Betaferon and Avonex are interferons that are proteins thought to help regulate the body's immune response against myelin. Adverse reactions include tissue loss at the injection site, flu-like symptoms, menstrual problems and depression. Betaferon comes with a warning from its distributor that mental disorders have been observed in patients who have used it. During a three-year study involving 372 patients, one suicide and four attempted suicides occurred. Although Avonex is reportedly easier to tolerate, it commonly causes flu-like symptoms, muscle aches, fever and chills. Copolymer-1 is a non-interferon drug, also thought to block myelin-specific autoimmune responses. Its side-effects include adverse tissue reactions at the injection site, chest pain, flushing, nausea, anxiety, weakness and painful joints. Reactions to all of these treatments are said to decrease over time but, for some patients, this has not been the case. In the US, the average cost of each of these medications is currently about $1,200 (£840) a month.

Many MS patients suffer painful muscle spasms. To combat these spasms, the FDA has approved dantrolene (Dantrium) and baclofen (Lioresal). Both are toxic substances that often cause serious side-effects. Many patients complain that they are generally ineffective in controlling muscle spasms. Doctors routinely prescribe tranquillizers, muscle relaxants and sedatives for muscle spasms. These drugs sometimes help control spasms but often leave patients in debilitated, dysfunctional states. These drugs are sometimes associated with hallucinations, and some patients have reported symptoms of withdrawal when discontinuing their use.

Today, a growing number of patients with multiple sclerosis who are discouraged by the lack of results from standard MS treatments are turning to marijuana as a sensible alternative. Many say marijuana gives them relief while avoiding the dangers and unwelcome side-effects of steroids, tranquillizers, muscle relaxants or sedatives. In the UK, ACT (Alliance for Cannabis Therapeutics) was formed by three MS sufferers who found that small amounts of cannabis were useful to help control the symptoms of MS. Thousands of MS sufferers in the UK are known to use the drug for medicinal reasons. The Multiple Sclerosis Society, which is represented in the current UK studies, is welcoming the research into the use of marijuana for the treatment of MS. They claim that marijuana is especially helpful in reducing their painful muscle spasms and tremors, and in regaining their muscle coordination and control. From their experience with long-term use, some MS patients believe that marijuana actually slows down the progression of their disease. They push aside the standard drugs that may make them feel worse and use marijuana in therapeutic doses that they feel are safer and more effective. If you have been diagnosed with MS, you may want to learn how other MS patients have used marijuana.

Bill Barrett, the glaucoma patient who told his story in Chapter 6, has also lived for 39 years with multiple sclerosis. Like many MS patients, Bill discovered the medicinal properties of marijuana after years of unsatisfactory treatment with standard therapies. Bill feels that marijuana has calmed his nerves and reduced the tightness in his legs. He also believes that marijuana has helped to relax him and that it has protected him from the stress that might trigger new attacks.

In April of 1958, I was misdiagnosed with polio. I remember that date because it was my mother's birthday, and I was twelve years old at the time. It began with a feeling of numbness in my legs. I didn't know what was wrong with me so I kept it a secret. Then, one day, my legs just stopped working.

At the hospital, the first thing they did was give me a spinal tap and then they diagnosed me with polio. I remained there in bed for three weeks during which they gave me some kind of treatment, placing hot rubber sheets all over my body. I don't know what exactly it was they were doing, but I remember how painful it was on my skin. They also gave me physical therapy, for which I returned to the hospital regularly during the first month after I left.

When I went back to school that semester, things were very different for me. I went through days having trouble using my legs. Even so, I tried to live as though nothing was wrong. Before graduating high school, I joined the Navy, but when I got to boot camp it became evident to me that I couldn't function normally with my legs. I could do all of the exercises we were given, but the marching, which we did so much of, was nearly impossible for me.

The problems with my legs persisted in this way until I had another attack about ten years ago. I was doing work on some machinery one day, and my body just collapsed. This time the numbness that began in my legs didn't stop at my waist. It went all the way up to my neck and into my arms. When it didn't stop at my armpits, I was afraid it was going to go into my face, but it didn't. It went all the way down my arms, and then paralysis set in. I lost feeling and movement in both my legs and arms.

I went through several doctors within four months, and none of them knew how to explain what was wrong with me. Then one day, after I took an MRI (Magnetic Resonance Imaging) scan, they informed me that I had multiple sclerosis, not polio. I had lived 29 years of my life wrongly thinking I had polio. Now, I didn't know who to trust, but it didn't seem I had many choices. At that point, I think they could've told me I had four months to live and I would have felt relieved.

Over the following years, I had a number of attacks and was kept on a regimen of many different medications. I've been prescribed nearly ten kinds of muscle relaxants to help me sleep, but none of them has ever really worked. I've been given other medications to stay awake. I've taken steroids, which were like speed. They were very hard to take because, unable to sleep or move around, all I could do was sit there after receiving the injections.

I know these steroids have hurt many people much more than they've helped them. They cause people to gain a lot of water weight in a short time, and it takes years to get rid of it. People are often hospitalized because of what these drugs do to their bodies, and they're placed at risk of cardiac arrest. When I took them, I became intensely frustrated and depressed. I grew angry at people, and my doctors felt I needed to be put on antidepressants.

After a while, I came to feel that I shouldn't take any more of the drugs they were giving me. None of them helped, and they seemed to be creating more problems for me than anything. So, I figured, with all the pharmaceuticals I was putting into my body, why not try something that other patients said really worked? Once I did, quite frankly, I felt marijuana was the only thing worth taking. It actually changed my condition entirely. It calmed my nerves and the tightness in my legs. This feeling is known to most MS patients as the 'girdle-effect.'

Marijuana also stopped the burning sensations I got in my feet. When I smoked it, I could feel an ease move throughout my limbs, and the pain would dissipate. I told my doctor about my marijuana use, and he told me that he didn't care what I used, as long as it was safe and it worked. He said he knew other patients who used it, too. About a year or two later, he gave me a letter stating that he would prescribe marijuana to me if it were legal, just as my ophthalmologist had done.

Since then, marijuana has been the only medicine I use regularly. I do currently have a prescription from my doctor for a light sleeping pill, but it just sits here. I feel that if I didn't use marijuana, I would be putting myself at risk of another attack. I would have pain and discomfort. I believe that, by keeping my system relaxed with marijuana, I won't have another attack.

I think there are many people who agree that marijuana works, but there is nothing they can do about it. I found I was even able to use marijuana while I was in the hospital in Detroit. Of course, I smoked it alone, quietly and discreetly, but I know the doctors could smell it when they walked in. They just looked at me and they never said a word.

The general attitude I get from other people with MS is, 'How do you do it?' To look at me you might not believe that I have MS, but follow me around all day and you will know. I was completely paralyzed ten years ago, and now I am able to sustain a normal life. My wheelchair sits in my garage now. I only use it if I have to go to the grocery store.

How could I let anybody change my life and make me go back to the miserable state I was in? What I'm doing has nothing to do with any drug problem in this country. I am dealing with a life-limiting medical condition, the best way I can. Given the alternatives, I don't know how anybody can tell me they wouldn't do the same for their health.

Stormy Ray has chronic-progressive multiple sclerosis, the most severe form. Seven years ago, when she was extremely debilitated, marijuana almost miraculously improved her condition. Stormy stopped taking her prescribed pharmaceuticals. Because marijuana was illegal, she began using the next best thing – Marinol. In the following account, Stormy explains why it has again become necessary for her to medicate with marijuana, despite the legal consequences.

My name is Stormy Ray and I'm a grandmother of four. There was a time when I would never have believed I'd be discussing marijuana. That's because this is not an avenue I have chosen. It was imposed on me. It's been imposed upon many others, too, our seniors and afflicted who, like me, cannot wait any longer for access to this stigmatized medicine.

Many people think the issue of medical marijuana is not important because they think it does not affect them. But, I ask, are you sure that it does not affect you? Your life may change someday, as mine did. Or you may find you have a loved one whose life suddenly depends on it.

I found out I had multiple sclerosis when I was 32. I was extremely healthy at the time, and I had a career running a successful insurance company. I wouldn't have suspected anything was wrong with me, until the day everything changed. I had just met with a client and I was walking back to my car. About half way there, my legs wouldn't take another step. All of a sudden, I could not walk anymore. In my three-piece suit, I sat down in the muddy street and crawled the rest of the way to my car. It was extremely difficult, but I managed to drive myself to a nearby hospital.

When I got there, the first physician I saw asked me if it was an emergency, and all I could tell him was that I couldn't walk. They immediately put me on pain relievers and took a series of X rays before my husband came and picked me up. From that day, it took eight months more of testing before they could tell me I had multiple sclerosis.

Within six months, I was bedridden and taking a load of pharmaceuticals. Unfortunately, these drugs weren't even a good Band-Aid for my symptoms. Steroids, like prednisone and ACTH, caused problems with my digestion and the ability to focus my eyes. The ACTH made my legs balloon up with fluid. I took it for only three or four days, but I puffed up immediately. Right now, I have a dear friend who's been taking these drugs, and she's now three times her normal size.

I was also taking many different medicines for the pain, including morphine, Valium (diazepam) and Flexeril (cyclobenzaprine hydrochloride). Some of these drugs were so ineffective that I would go into the hospital for a 100-milligram shot of Demerol (meperidine or pethidine) and, because it wouldn't work, they would have to give me 100 milligrams more before I left. I would leave like a zombie and then, shortly after getting home, the pain would return.

By 1991, I was actually dying. The pharmaceuticals were interacting badly, and my system was shutting down. My doctor didn't think I was going to make it. By this time, I had to be taken to the hospital every three days for shots of Demerol (pethidine) and morphine. But, the shots never took away the sharpness of my pain. I was in indescribable agony and my ligaments were severely curled. They were drawn up at my knees, my elbows, and my ankles. I believe this occurs because the disease prevents vital messages from going to and from your brain. You lose not only control, but a certain awareness in places in your body. I had reached this point and there was nothing I could do.

One evening, a close friend came over to our home with a joint and told me how he thought it could help me. Even though it was illegal, I wanted to try it because nothing else had given me any hope. When I did, what happened in my body was truly amazing. It wasn't so much a rush I felt, as a different awareness moving throughout my body. I took about two or three hits and, almost immediately, it was as if parts of me were being turned on again. It allowed me to relax in a way that I hadn't been able to do since I first became sick. It made me feel as if I was wrapped up in a blanket, warm and comfortable. I wouldn't have thought anything could give me such relief.

My husband and I felt we weren't the type of people that could go out on the street and obtain marijuana, so we looked for something that was legal. We searched for a doctor who would prescribe Marinol. I did eventually find one, but he wasn't able to tell me what dosage I should take. I had to figure it out for myself, and it took about two weeks of trial and error. I found that one capsule every four hours worked best. Within 24 hours of taking my first pill, the three-month-old migraine headache I'd had simply went away. It was as if I was above my pain looking down at it, rather than being in the middle of it. After a few months, I threw out all the other pharmaceuticals I had, and I've continued using only Marinol since then.

There are some problems with Marinol, though. It's expensive and it does more to hinder than help some people. I know people who have found it debilitating. But after taking the number of heavy pharmaceuticals that I have, it doesn't affect me that way. People don't realize how the other drugs can put you in 'la la land,' a lot more so than Marinol.

Also, if you have an exacerbation, it can take a while to get relief with Marinol. It doesn't have that same overall body flush as marijuana. But the main problem for me has been that, after a while, your body builds up a tolerance, and Marinol loses its effectiveness. I've noticed that it isn't working for me the same way it used to. One pill used to work for a little less than four hours, and now it only works for about two hours.

So now, I find myself in a rather frustrating position. As Marinol becomes less and less effective, my need for legal and accessible marijuana becomes clear and urgent. I know from my past experience that it works. Should I have to curl back up in pain because it is illegal? I don't want to go back to the way I was, but I'm not a criminal, and I shouldn't have to be forced into acting like one to be well. No one should have to risk getting arrested to get their medicine.

I don't think it would be that way if people had a better understanding. Marijuana in its natural form is one of the safest, most therapeutic substances in the world. We're not talking a Band-Aid. Marijuana works because it allows those vital messages to go through to different parts of your body – the parts that the disease seems to take away from you. In this position, people like me find it becomes a matter of doing what any sane person would do. We use marijuana to be well and there isn't anything criminal about that.

In clinical tests, synthetic THC has decreased the severity of muscle spasm associated with multiple sclerosis. Many American MS patients use synthetic THC, or Marinol, even though their doctors cannot legally prescribe it, because it provides more relief than other pharmaceuticals. (In the US, Marinol can only be legally prescribed for the side-effects of cancer chemotherapy and AIDS wasting syndrome.)

In the UK, Cesamet (Nabilone) is currently licensed as an anti-emetic for chemotherapy patients, but doctors can prescribe the cannabinoid for MS sufferers on a 'named patient' basis. Up to a quarter of all MS sufferers may be using marijuana, either in its prescribed form, or in its natural state, often with the approval of their doctors. However, Marinol's therapeutic effects occasionally diminish as patients develop a tolerance for it. This tolerance does not seem to occur with marijuana. Like Stormy Ray, such patients find it necessary to supplement their Marinol use with marijuana. Others who try Marinol have a difficult time achieving the proper dose without intolerable psychological side-effects, and they prefer using only marijuana.

Reports that MS patients were using marijuana to successfully treat their symptoms prompted research on synthetic THC in the late 1970s. Dr Carl Ellenberger in New York heard from several MS patients that marijuana relieved the stiffness in their legs and aided their ability to walk. Examining these patients before and after they smoked marijuana, he found their claims to be valid. In 1978, along with his colleague, Dr Denis Petro, Ellenberger requested permission from the Drug Enforcement Administration (DEA) to launch a controlled study of the effects of THC on human spasticity. The DEA refused them permission to use marijuana for the study but, instead, gave them permission to use synthetic THC (Petro, 1981).

Their research results supported Dr Ellenberger's earlier observations. All nine participating patients showed significant reduction in spasticity with THC, suggesting further study was warranted. A few factors, however, led Petro and Ellenberger to conclude that synthetic THC was not the ideal drug for treating spasticity. The therapeutic effects of synthetic THC seemed to diminish after repeated use, as patients developed a tolerance to it. Most of the patients reported that they didn't like taking THC, and they preferred smoking marijuana. The same patients showed clear improvement after using marijuana.

One drawback of Marinol is the difficulty in achieving the right dose. Another may be that THC, in the absence of the other compounds found in marijuana smoke, is not sufficient for treating spasticity. Researchers believe that cannabidiol, one of the other 460 known compounds found in marijuana, may work more effectively than THC. Animal studies have shown that THC in high doses can actually excite the muscles. Cannabidiol is thought to counteract this effect (Rosenthal, 1997; 39).

We need more research on marijuana and the many compounds found within it. This would provide a better understanding of just how marijuana can aid the treatment of multiple sclerosis. Generally, it is used for treating spasticity and pain. However, there are many different symptoms that afflict people with MS, and there may be other ways in which marijuana is therapeutic.

Another potential use of marijuana, not yet thoroughly explored, is in the treatment of ataxia, which is the loss of muscle coordination. This possibility offers hope to MS patients who are debilitated by ataxia. In the last ten years, a few small clinical studies discussing the effect of marijuana on ataxia have been published in neurology journals (Grinspoon, 1997; 87). More recently, receptor sites for marijuana have been discovered in areas of the brain that control memory, cognition, pain, nausea and motor coordination. This finding supports the notion that marijuana may somehow facilitate transmission of nerve impulses from the brain to the muscles to improve symptoms in MS. It is interesting that no marijuana receptors are found in areas of the brain that control breathing and heart activity which may explain why no one has ever died of a marijuana overdose.

There are claims that marijuana not only relieves the symptoms of multiple sclerosis, but also treats the progression of the disease itself. Some scientists believe that marijuana has potential to both enhance and suppress immune responses. Though its suppressing tendencies are thought to be mild, they are of concern to doctors in the treatment of AIDS. For treating an autoimmune disease like MS, on the other hand, researchers see promising possibilities.

A recent report by a National Institutes of Health panel has pointed to the need for further research on the immune-modulating potential of marijuana. Much of the available evidence comes from animal studies. In one late 1980s study, guinea pigs were exposed to an infection similar to MS known as experimental autoimmune encephalomyelitis (EAE). The guinea pigs that received THC resisted the infection, with either mild or no symptoms. More than 95 per cent of them survived. In contrast, all the guinea pigs treated with a placebo developed severe EAE, and more than 98 per cent of them died. Reduced inflammation was also found in the animals treated with THC (Grinspoon, 1997; 94).

Regardless of the positions taken by medical societies and government officials on the issue of medical marijuana, it is becoming a more popular choice for thousands of MS sufferers. Patients who use it say they simply know that it works because of their own observations. Often, they have had to experiment on their own to find the proper dose, since there is no medically established treatment using marijuana. This can be difficult at first, but it is possible with a little trial and error. If you have MS and the available MS treatments have not worked for you, you may want to try using marijuana to relieve your symptoms. Unfortunately, you may feel considerable stress due to the illegal status of medical marijuana. Many patients know of that stress and feel that it can put them in danger of another attack, relapse or exacerbation.

Fortunately, in almost every country there are support

groups – made up of patients, doctors and healthcare advocates – formed to share information about MS treatments and other aspects of the disease. Many of these groups are becoming increasingly active and vocal about a patient's right to use medical marijuana, such as ACT in the UK. You may want to seek out one of these groups for more information about your rights should you decide that marijuana is the right medicine for you.

Chapter 8
Paraplegia and Quadriplegia

When spinal cord illness or injury leads to paralysis, it is often accompanied by painful and uncontrollable muscle spasms. Many patients with this problem have turned to marijuana for relief. Paraplegia occurs when the spinal cord injury or disease affects the middle or lower half of the spinal cord. This results in weakness or paralysis in the lower half of the body. When the injury is higher on the spinal cord, close to the neck, the weakness or paralysis affects the arms as well as the lower body. This condition is called quadriplegia. Multiple sclerosis, discussed in the last chapter, can also lead to either paraplegia or quadriplegia.

It is a common mistake to think that patients with paraplegia and quadriplegia have lost all movement in their limbs. Actually, they have only lost conscious control over such movement. In these types of paralyses, there is a loss of both sensation and control of muscle movement. Nonetheless, the muscles can still move involuntarily, as they do in muscle spasms. These spasms are often severe and can cause injury to the muscles or bones. In addition, spasms can cause pain in other parts of the body and often result in loss of sleep. Doctors call the condition of severe, recurrent spasms caused by nerve damage spasticity.

As we mentioned in Chapter 7 regarding multiple sclerosis, there were two drugs specifically designed to control spasticity: dantrolene (Dantrium) and baclofen (Lioresal). These drugs can be highly toxic. Potential risks include developing inflammation of the liver (hepatitis), stomach ulcers with bleeding, constipation, anorexia, abdominal cramps, speech disturbances, seizures, visual distortions, erratic blood pressure, mental confusion, clinical depression, kidney disturbances, feelings of suffocation and, possibly, death. It is important to keep toxicity of more standard medicines in mind when thinking about the potential dangers of marijuana.

Doctors also prescribe other muscle relaxants, sedatives and tranquillizers such as meprobamate, diazepam (Valium), phenobarbitone, chloropromazine (Chloractil or Largactil), or similar drugs to control spasticity. Some patients find that these drugs do little to relieve their spasms and have undesirable short- and long-term side-effects. They can be addictive and are capable of causing damage to the stomach, liver, kidneys and digestive system. Some patients who use them complain of depression. An extreme solution to the problem of muscle spasms is to surgically remove nerve tissue in the spinal cord that activates muscle contractions. This procedure eliminates the spasms and their painful effects, but in doing so, it creates other long-term problems. Though the muscles no longer spasm, they do lose tone and eventually atrophy, or wither away due to the lack of use and activity.

The fact that marijuana can control muscle spasms has been known for a very long time, even in ancient China. In the 19th century, Scotsman Dr W. B. O'Shaughnessy observed marijuana being used for this purpose in India. He wrote several papers describing marijuana in the treatment of the severe muscle spasms (spasticity) associated with tetanus, rabies and other diseases. O'Shaughnessy recorded the reduction or elimination of severe spasticity without harmful effects. Many of his observations were printed in a report issued by the Ohio State Medical Society in 1860. In the late 19th century, the personal physician of Queen Victoria, Dr J. R. Reynolds, reported using marijuana to treat muscle spasms, epilepsy and migraines.

In recent times, there has been no scientifically controlled research looking at the effect of marijuana on the control of the muscle spasms caused by spinal cord injuries. However, there have been a few published observations and informal studies. More research is warranted. In a 1974 survey of ten male patients with spinal cord injuries, eight reported experiencing muscle spasms. Of the eight, five claimed that marijuana decreased their spasticity (Dunn, 1974). Since then, other surveys have suggested that about half of the patients with spinal cord injuries can probably use marijuana to control their muscle spasms. In 1990, Swiss neurologists reported studying one paraplegic who showed significant improvement when THC was used in the treatment of his pain, muscle spasms, quality of sleep and bladder control (Grinspoon, 1997; 100).

Bobby Steele, a well-known musician, is a patient with paraplegia who was unable to get satisfactory relief from prescribed drugs. As a result, he self-medicated with marijuana and was able to achieve significant improvement.

I was born with spina bifida. That's a 99 per cent fatal birth defect in which the spinal cord is exposed or protrudes from the spinal column. I wasn't even aware that I had it until, one day, when I was eight years old, some other kids noticed the scar on my back when we were swimming.

Growing up I didn't have many problems until I was around ten years old. My left leg began turning outward, and my foot began dragging when I walked. By the time I was 12 years old, I had weakness in my left leg, and both legs seemed to stop growing. My doctors tried to correct this with physical therapy and surgery on my foot, but it never really helped.

When I was around 13, my parents noticed that I wasn't standing up straight after sitting for long periods of time. When they questioned me about it, I explained that it was painful for me to do so. So they took me back to the doctor, and he discovered I had developed a cyst on the base of my spinal cord, most likely from the residual tissue of my spinal cord at birth. I underwent surgery that year to remove the cyst at Columbia Presbyterian in New York City.

After the procedure, I was able to make it out of the hospital with the aid of a cane and a brace, but I was essentially paralyzed from the waist down. I couldn't coordinate any movement in my legs, but I felt occasional, uncontrollable twitches in them. For a while, I had to use crutches to move around. Eventually, I did regain feeling and movement in my right leg, but my left leg remained partially paralyzed.

By early 1986, I was having such violent spasms in my legs, I went for weeks without sleep. The specialist I saw gave me Flexeril (cyclobenzaprine hydrochloride), which did absolutely nothing for my spasms. Then I started taking Carisoma (carisoprodol). It worked for about a month, until I built up a resistance to it. Then they were going to put me on double doses. I didn't want to go along with that, so I stopped taking it entirely.

At some point they gave me Dilaudid (hydromorphone), a dangerous opiate narcotic that has been known to lead to heroin use for people who become addicted to it. Taking these drugs, I was still having violent spasms, but I was constantly stoned. After a while, they would inevitably stop working, and my dosages would increase. Eventually, I objected to continuing treatment with these drugs, because I felt like I was becoming an addict.

Then, one day, I was at a friend's house and he broke out a joint. When I got home that night, I looked at my girlfriend in amazement and I told her that my legs felt fine. Then I went to sleep. I tried it a few more times to be sure it was, in fact, the marijuana that was having this effect on me. Then I went to the hospital and told my doctors what I had discovered.

My healthcare providers ridiculed me, but my family and close friends understood. My parents even made an 'about-face' in regard to their views about my smoking. They have come to feel that there is something seriously wrong with the way marijuana is stigmatized, when a seriously ill or debilitated person who is helped by marijuana can be harassed or even imprisoned for it.

Before I used marijuana, I was in and out of the hospital with sore throats, bronchitis and colds. My spasms interrupted my sleep so regularly that my immune system was weakened. But once I started using marijuana for my spasms, my overall health improved remarkably. When I ran into one of the nurses from the hospital, at the post office, she recognized me and asked why I hadn't been in for a long time. I told her that once I started smoking pot, I was able to sleep and I stopped having so many problems with my health. She saw that I was better, and she acknowledged the sensibility of it.

I only smoke marijuana at night, when it's time to go to bed. At other times, if I feel spasms in my legs, I take two or three puffs and they go away. I know that according to modern medicine, there isn't enough official evidence to substantiate our claims about marijuana. But that doesn't matter when you find something that really works without making you feel like you're harming your body. Too many people, including doctors, have seen positive results with medical marijuana to ignore or discount their experiences.

In 1987, I was in the hospital for foot surgery. When I had the opportunity, I went outside to smoke some marijuana. A doctor walked by and he looked at me. As he passed, he said it was the best medicine. He knew that. I know that, too, and so do many, many other people who use it to be well.

Tony Leger used marijuana to maintain his health without debilitating side-effects for most of his adult life. Eventually, he faced legal prosecution for his use of medical marijuana, and as a result, he could no longer medicate. At that point, his health degenerated into a paraplegic state. This is Tony's story:

I am a 36-year-old husband, father, businessman and veteran of the US Navy. No one can pin the title 'druggie' on me, and I have found that there are a lot of other people like me. They use marijuana for conditions they have been forced to live with.

I have a degenerative disc disease that mimics arthritic pain. Mobility has become a big issue in my life. Pain management has become addiction management because of the pharmaceuticals I've had to take. This is all compounded by the existence of two cysts in my spinal cord cavity, where I have a protruding node that's caused by a genetic disorder, known as Schmorl's node. Because of the cysts, bloating has become a factor in my health.

But the biggest issue with both of these conditions is inflammation. Because of the inflammation that occurs in my spinal cord cavity, I get tremors in the calves of my legs. It starts with little tremors that create a rippling effect on the surface of my skin. Pretty soon, numbness sets in, and then the reflexes in my right leg go away. My motor coordination fails and I begin to limp. Within a few weeks, I can't walk, and I can't feel when my feet hit the floor, because I've lost almost all sensation in the bottom of my feet.

I was 17 years old when the first signs that something was wrong appeared. As a wrestler in high school, I had injuries that wouldn't heal. They left me with a slight, nagging muscle strain, and an intense tightening in my back. When I went to see a doctor, my X rays showed no outward signs of any problem. Since I didn't know anything was wrong with me, I just sort of dealt with the pain as a teenager.

Then, when I started using marijuana recreationally, I noticed that it made my back feel better. My parents were also divorcing at the time, and smoking marijuana seemed to lift some of my depression.

Though I had all these physical conditions early on, they never caused me any real problems until two years ago, in November of 1995. My wife, Lindsay, and I were raided by a drug task force. They found three marijuana plants in pharmaceutical grow boxes. We were charged with felony manufacturing of a controlled substance, felony possession and felony intent to distribute. We were also put into a urinalysis program in which we were subject to daily testing.

I would say that at that time my health was at 95 per cent, and I had no debilitation. But because I could no longer use marijuana medically, I went to the doctors to be put on some sort of replacement treatment. That's when my health began to take a turn for the worse. I was prescribed an opiate called Vicodin (a combination of hydrocodone and paracetamol) for acute pain, a muscle relaxant called Flexeril (cyclobenzaprine), a pain reliever called Ultram (tramadol) and ibuprofen.

I started out taking these drugs as directed. They had me on 3600 milligrams a day of ibuprofen. It helped me with the pain from the inflammation, but it badly affected my mobility because it caused me to retain fluid. When I told my doctors, they increased the Vicodin, which I continued to take with the Flexeril and the Ultram.

The Ultram was dangerous, and I had too many problems

with it. After my third day of taking it, it made my voice change and I began to have flu-like symptoms. So I stopped taking it, and I went back to taking ibuprofen. I actually had withdrawals from the Ultram. My body would begin shaking and I'd break out into a sweat. Then, because they didn't want me taking high doses of ibuprofen, they put me on Naprosyn (naproxen). This worked well for a while, but it made me feel real 'dingy,' and after a little more than a week, I broke out in skin rashes. The truth is, marijuana was the only thing that worked without problems like this.

I went into custody January 4, 1997. Before going to the jail, I went to see the doctor to make sure I had all my medications, which the judge in the courtroom said I should have access to. But once I got to jail, the medical staff wouldn't let me have them. Within two weeks I could no longer walk. I could stand up, but I didn't have any movement control. My cellmate was bringing me my food.

I stayed this way for the rest of my 38 days. At one point, a guard reported to a nurse that I needed help, and the nurse came to see me. When he learned that I was a veteran of the US Navy, he told me he would try to release my medication during the weekend when he was there. Come Monday, he said, the other staff would probably restrict them from me once again. He was only able to access the Ultram (tramadol) and the Aleve (naproxen) but, once I took these medicines, I felt an immediate improvement because they eased the pain. At the end of my 38 days, I left the jail in a paraplegic state. While I had some ability to move my feet, I'd lost almost all feeling and motor control in both my legs.

After I was released, I went to see my doctor and he was not happy. The last time he'd seen me, I was able to get around using a cane. He immediately put me back on my medications. I had picked up a head cold in custody, and as it began to diminish, I developed symptoms of Bell's palsy. This causes muscle weakness on one side of my face so that it appears that I have a drooping eyelid. I don't know if it was the cold or the condition of my health in custody that brought it on. When I went back to see my doctor, he was unavailable, so I was referred to another doctor.

As soon as this doctor walked into the room and saw me, I could tell by the look on his face that he was disturbed. He thought the types of symptoms I had were unusual for a degenerative disc disease. He said he thought they were rather indicative of a spinal cord injury. He requested that I have an MRI scan taken immediately.

Up to this point, my doctors thought my problems were caused by inflamed scar tissue that was restricting flow from the nerve conduit. Other than offering that opinion, they couldn't explain what was causing my numbness or my problems with mobility. They seemed puzzled, but they never explored it.

The MRI scan revealed that I had two cysts and a protruding node, referred to as a Schmorl's node. This was located along my spine, inside the spinal cord cavity. The only other thing the neurologist told me about it was that I was not a candidate for surgery. For the first time, it became apparent to me that they were considering the possibility. They explained to me that the amount of scar tissue that would form with a surgical removal would likely cause more harm than good.

I told them that I didn't think I would agree to surgery anyway because I knew a much better way to deal with the problem. I told them about my marijuana use. They were quite uncomfortable with this information, however they seemed to rely on my experience for understanding. I told them that once I no longer faced the legal situation I was in, they wouldn't be seeing my face again.

In June of 1997, I went back into custody. Four days before my probation was to expire, which would've been June 16, I was summoned into court. Violations that had been set aside previously were again brought up against me. While I had been in custody in January, my wife had submitted an article in a local Vancouver paper called *The Columbian*. She explained our situation and that I was not receiving my medication. We filed a federal lawsuit because all other avenues of redress had failed.

When the judge put me into custody, I informed him that I had filed a federal suit for the withholding of my medical treatment, and that numbers of people were looking at my case this time. He ordered that my medical treatment be taken care of during my custody. I went into custody on June 12. On June 14, the doctor called me and signed a form giving me authorization to receive ibuprofen. It wasn't until nearly a week later, on June 19, that I receive my first dose.

On June 20, I reported my lack of medical treatment to my court-appointed attorney. I also mentioned to him that I didn't think I should still be in custody. My probation was set to expire on June 16, and as far as I was aware, I never received any notification that the proper paperwork had been filed to freeze my probation time while in custody. He said he didn't know anything about this, but he would look into it.

On the night of June 23, a guard came in and announced that I was to be released. No one could tell me what was going on. I was assisted by other inmates who helped me gather my things and then helped me get through the doors to be released. From the doors, I was helped by a guard outside to the pay phone where I called home to my wife.

The next morning I went to my scheduled hearing and was informed that my case had been removed from the docket. Before I could even figure out what questions to ask, the next case was called up. I just stood there as the charge of child rape in the third degree was read. Then the prosecutor requested that the defendant be booked and released. There ended any hope I'd had in our criminal justice system.

When I got home, after I came out of shock, I probably cried for about two hours. I couldn't talk for a while. After I was able to resurrect myself, I called my probation officer who could not tell me a thing about what had happened to my case. She said, as far as she knew, I was still supposed to be in jail. I told her I wanted to know what happened to my due process and, to this day, I have not heard a word back from her.

On July 20, I was told that my attorney received a call from the prosecutor's office informing him that my charges had been removed from the docket, and there would be no further court hearings. He advised me that I still needed to pay the fines I owed. It was not until August that I was able to get my hands on any paperwork. I found out that the Department of Corrections had not had the authority to hold me in custody past the end of my probation. I went to the prosecutor's office myself for an official explanation, which I did not get, and to retrieve some of my property. To this day, I have received neither of these things, and I have not heard a word from the prosecutor who assured me that he would follow up with me.

I believe that every time they violated my civil rights, they also violated the civil rights of every citizen in this country. From what I've been through, I can see that there is a major degeneration of our system of justice, and drug prohibition is a major cause of it. After I was released from custody in June, I went back to medicating with marijuana. By the end of August, I could essentially reduce my intake of the pharmaceuticals to only a few weeks. The recurrence and severity of my spasms have been significantly reduced.

In August, I went to see a doctor who is very familiar with

the medical usefulness of marijuana. I was referred to him by an old college friend of his. He gave me a written recommendation for marijuana and he gave me a prescription for Marinol. I have found that Marinol is a good antidepressant and it's a good pain reliever. Unfortunately, Marinol has not aided my mobility. It doesn't free up the stiffness and the binding of my muscles the way marijuana does. The most valuable thing Marinol does is remove the legal stigma. Who can say that marijuana is not medicine when the Food and Drug Administration promote Marinol, which is synthetic THC?

I continue to medicate with marijuana because it's most effective, and I substitute my use with Marinol when I have to. My mobility is getting closer to 90 per cent, and I'm almost back to the level of health I was at before all this legal hassle began. I'm back to leading off with my right foot when I walk and I no longer drag on my right side.

The fact that I have been willing to risk so much, should show that I am 100 per cent certain marijuana is the only medicine that is going to bring me the relief I need. I believe I can take it for the rest of my life without jeopardizing my ability to be a husband to my wife, a father to my two children, and to show even one person who suffers with spinal cord injury or illness that there is hope, and a way to live.

There is a great deal of anecdotal evidence, like this moving account, that supports the claim that marijuana is of particular use to paraplegics and quadriplegics. Tragically, the most common source of such stories are the thousands of paralysed veterans of the war in Vietnam, many of whom are treated in Veterans Administration (VA) hospitals across the US. When one of us (RB) first encountered patients using marijuana, it was in the cancer wards during an internal medicine residency at the Portland VA Hospital in Oregon. It was common knowledge among doctors and patients there that marijuana could relieve the nausea caused by chemotherapy.

One evening, while on call and exploring the hospital, he entered the rehabilitation ward, where a group of Vietnam veterans with various levels of paraplegia were using marijuana. Most of them had begun to smoke marijuana in Vietnam. After being paralysed, they had found that marijuana helped their leg spasms and their pain. It didn't seem to cause them as many undesirable side-effects as the medicines their doctors were giving them. At a VA clinic, there was an amputee who had been badly maimed by a land mine and had lost both of his legs. Marijuana helped him with his phantom limb pain, a phenomenon experienced when people lose limbs or parts of their body. The limb is no longer there, but the nerves in the brain that controlled the limb are, and they create the sensation of pain.

Many doctors and nurses who have worked with paraplegics and quadriplegics have witnessed marijuana being used therapeutically. However, given the legal situation, most don't like to talk about it. Nonetheless, there is an understanding among these health care professionals that marijuana use deserves to be quietly recommended or at least tolerated in patients with varying degrees of spasticity associated with the paralysis that accompanies spinal cord illnesses and injuries. It is reasonable to expect that this will continue until modern medicine is able to offer a safer, more effective treatment.

Chapter 9
Epilepsy

Epilepsy is a persistent (chronic) condition of the brain. It involves unpredictable abnormal electrical discharges or misfirings of brain cells (neurons). This misfiring in the brain can cause episodes of bodily convulsions, loss of coordination, loss of consciousness or altered sensory states. These episodes are commonly called seizures. People with epilepsy have persistent and recurring seizures. One may be born with epilepsy, or may acquire it as a result of disease or injury.

Epileptic seizures are commonly classified as partial seizures or generalized seizures. Partial seizures are more common and start in an isolated part of the brain. Partial seizures can be described as either simple or complex. When a simple partial seizure occurs, a person retains consciousness. The person with epilepsy may experience uncontrollable twitching or stiffening in a limb. There may be a tingling sensation, a change in consciousness or an odd smell without a source. The subjective sensations that may warn of an impending event are called an 'aura'.

Complex partial seizures cause an impairment of consciousness. During this type of seizure, a person may act confused, aimless, fidgety, emotional or disturbed. They are likely to have no memory of the event after it is over. A simple partial seizure may progress to a complex partial seizure and then become a generalized seizure as the abnormal electrical discharge spreads to the entire brain.

Generalized seizures thus involve abnormal discharges or misfirings in all regions of the brain and result in impairment of consciousness. Behaviour during generalized seizures may range from a blank stare with little or no movement (petit mal or 'absence' seizures) to dramatic bodily convulsions (grand mal seizures). During these convulsions, the patient may have difficulty breathing and turn blue. They may also bite their tongue and may lose control of urine or stool. When they regain consciousness, they do not remember the event and are very sleepy.

Epilepsy is treated with a class of drugs called anticonvulsants. Standard drugs in this class include carbamazepine (Tegretol), phenytoin (Epantin or Pentran), primidone (Mysoline), clonazepam (Rivotril), ethosuximide (Zarontin) and phenobarbitone. Newer drugs are coming onto the market but there is less experience using them. Doctors prescribe anticonvulsant or antiepileptic drugs according to the types of seizures patients experience and how well the patient can tolerate the drugs. Many patients have a poor response to these drugs, even when they are taken in combination.

In addition to problems with effectiveness, there can be serious side-effects resulting from the use of anticonvulsants. While these side-effects do not always occur, they can include nausea, headaches, loss of hair, swelling of gum tissue, impotence, depression, poor coordination (ataxia), liver failure, depressed blood counts and even psychosis.

Some people with grand mal seizures say they can prevent their seizures entirely by smoking marijuana. Others, who suffer complex partial seizures, report that marijuana also curbs their symptoms and prevents loss of consciousness. Marijuana is not considered useful for treating petit mal or absence seizures and may even worsen them.

In response to mounting anecdotal evidence that marijuana

can help at least some people with epilepsy, patients are experimenting with its use. Some are finding that marijuana works in conjunction with the prescribed drugs they are taking. Others find that marijuana works best for them when it is used without other drugs. Either way, these epileptic patients have made marijuana a necessary part of their medical treatment.

Valerie Corral coordinates a medical marijuana cooperative in Santa Cruz, California. It's called the Wo-Men's Alliance for Medical Marijuana (WAMM). Valerie sustained injuries in a car accident in 1973 that left her with epilepsy. She used the standard anticonvulsant drugs to treat it, but soon found that she could no longer tolerate the side-effects. At that time, Valerie discovered that marijuana could control her seizures.

> I was a university student and a sculptor when I suffered injuries from a serious car accident in 1973. It was then that I became an epileptic. Epilepsy changed my plans for the future. I had to drop out of school. It also changed the way I perceived the world around me.
>
> Because of the pharmaceuticals I took, I wound up in a complete drug stupor. I took antiepilepsy drugs, like Epantin or Pentran (phenytoin) and Mysoline (primidone). But no matter how my doctors varied the combination, or the dosage, I remained in the same epileptic state. For pain, I took Percodan (a combination of oxycodone and aspirin) and Valium (diazepam). On these drugs, I became overwhelmingly disconnected, isolated and alone. I was paranoid. My personality changed. By the end of that first year, I was in a deep depression.
>
> Instead of adding something to my health and my life, these so-called medicines had taken so much away from me. When I hear anyone argue that marijuana can't be used as medicine because of the psychoactive effect it can have, I

know they have never had to take these pharmaceuticals and experience their far more severe psychoactive effects.

For about six months, I was taking birth control pills while on these medications, because I didn't want to get pregnant. Then my husband, Mike, read in the *Physicians Desk Reference* that the drugs I was taking, in combination, can cause water on the brain. I got so scared that I quit taking everything – cold turkey. This was extremely dangerous, as I would find out. My seizure activity increased. When I took one of the old pills again the seizures stopped, so I resumed taking the pills.

In the meantime, Mike had read about the medicinal properties of marijuana. I remember how I felt after the first time I tried it. The intensity of my aura became diluted, and the inevitable shaking never came. It surprised the hell out of me. I thought nothing that simple could actually work when I had tried everything modern science and medicine could offer. But marijuana did work. I kept saying to myself, 'How can this be?'

Marijuana became my regular medicine. I took it with the other drugs, which I planned to gradually wean myself from. When I discussed my experience with my doctors and nurses, I don't think they believed me. At least, at first. But they gave me their tacit approval. I think they did so because they knew so little about the cause and origin of seizures. They were willing to look at anything that can reduce the onset or the trigger.

It's important for us, as patients, to change our view of doctors. [In the US] we pay our doctors, and then we forget they're our employees. If the plumber leaves your house, and the toilet doesn't work, we call her back. We ask doctors to save our lives, and then we become complacent in our treatment, because we want them to do just that. We want to believe we'll be cured. Once we accept that position, we give up control. When our treatments don't work, we think there isn't anything more we can do.

Until the mid-1970s, epileptics were often admitted into institutions. Epilepsy was treated as a mental illness. But it's not. It's a physical disorder. So we're only talking about 20 years of treating the disorder for what it is. Not everything is known about the possibilities for our treatment.

Eventually, I was able to stop taking all of my prescription drugs, though it took me a little more than two years to do so. I decreased my amounts, slowly and cautiously, always keeping a rolled joint with me in case I felt a seizure coming on.

I've been able to control my epilepsy for over 20 years now with marijuana. I no longer feel cut off from my life, as I did before. I always keep a certain level of marijuana in my body, and that's what prevents me from having seizures. When I do have an aura, which is an early premonition or manifestation of a seizure, I use marijuana immediately and the feeling goes away. My auras now serve as little indicators. They give me enough time to sit down and take a few hits of marijuana in order to prevent a seizure.

I still have problems, so it's important for me to keep some marijuana available to treat them. Sometimes I get massive headaches. When I use marijuana, it puts a veil between me and my pain. If I don't use marijuana, because I get tired of medicating, my problems and seizure onsets increase.

I don't believe Marinol would help me because using THC alone is not the safest, nor the most effective way, to treat seizures. Plus, why should I have to pay $600 (£420) a month for THC when I can grow marijuana myself and get a better form of THC for free? Marijuana works for me. I don't think anyone who's lived with something like epilepsy would quit using medicine that's really working in order to take something else.

When my grandmother was sick with leukemia in 1974, we told her about marijuana. She thought it was immoral and unladylike for a woman to smoke, so we put it in teas for her. But once she felt the benefits, she changed her mind, and she eventually smoked it. You see, no matter what you think, your experience might change.

No, I don't believe marijuana is a panacea. I don't think it's going to change the world, and that isn't the point. I am not just an epileptic, and I'm not just someone who supports the medical use of marijuana. I'm a gardener, and a researcher, and someone who works with people who are dying. For people who are really sick, good medicine can change their sense of dying, to an attitude and a possibility of living. Marijuana works in that way. Marijuana is good medicine.

For ten years, Alan Martinez relied on marijuana to prevent his grand mal seizures. In 1986, he discovered that the mind-numbing phenobarbitone he regularly took to control his epilepsy could be put aside. A neurologist recommended that he try marijuana. When he did, he found that a few hits on a marijuana cigarette prevented his seizures with no debilitating side-effects. He also discovered that he could get the therapeutic effect without smoking enough to even get high.

The smoking changed Alan's life – from dependence to independence. Lacking financial resources, he started training as a nurse's aide. Once qualified he accepted a variety of assignments, focusing on those in greatest need, patients with terminal cancer and AIDS, and elderly people unable to care for themselves. He also met other epileptics who had made the same discovery about marijuana that he had.

To get his medicine, Alan had to make his purchases on the streets. He was not comfortable, so he did what many patients in his predicament do. He started growing his own marijuana.

At the time, he lived a quiet life with his partner in their home in Santa Rosa, California. Nevertheless, growing marijuana is a crime, even if you are doing it to medicate yourself. A neighbour saw five marijuana seedlings growing in Alan's kitchen window and turned him in. He was charged with felony cultivation, for which he faced up to three years in prison.

That's when one of us (BZ) met Alan. It was the summer of 1996, when Alan was under indictment awaiting trial. The political campaign to pass Proposition 215, the California initiative to decriminalize the medical use of marijuana, needed public advocates. Leaders of the campaign had heard about Alan's case and thought he would be a good example to put before California voters. Reporters were anxious to question him. Alan flew down to Los Angeles to prepare for their questions. A full-dress press conference on a controversial subject is a very difficult task for an inexperienced spokesperson, but Alan was willing to try.

As this usually shy and reserved man stepped in front of the microphones, he was suddenly transformed. He spoke in compelling, emotional and descriptive language. He was passionate, and it became clear that he had found his public voice. Even the hard-bitten LA reporters were visibly moved by his story. Alan explained to them that he had used marijuana for ten years, and that with it, he was not only able to completely control his seizures, but that in the process he had become a productive member of society, as well.

In the following months, Alan spoke on behalf of the Proposition 215 campaign on several occasions. But his public appearances cost him his job. His employers didn't want a 'pothead' emptying their patients' bedpans. His loss only strengthened his resolve. He became more assertive and self-confident. He had a lot riding on the outcome of the election. If Proposition 215 won, cultivation of marijuana by a medical patient would no longer be a crime.

The decisive victory for Proposition 215 in November 1996 made a lot of people happy, none more than Alan. He looked forward to his preliminary hearing in December, confident that all charges against him would be dismissed. Unfortunately, he was naïve. The judge, bending to the turbo-charged politics of the 'War on Drugs', ignored the will of California voters and ruled that Alan would have to stand trial.

Many months were then consumed by hearings and appeals. During that time, Alan no longer felt comfortable using marijuana. He feared the implications of a second brush with the law. So he gave it up. The price was high. His seizures returned. On 3 July 1997, Alan was killed in a one-car accident while driving alone on a back road. He apparently had a seizure behind the wheel. He was 41 years old.

The anticonvulsant properties of marijuana may be the oldest of its known medical benefits. Marijuana was used as a medicine for epilepsy by ancient societies in China, Africa, India, Greece and Rome. Written testimonies of its usefulness, such as the aforementioned one by Dr W. B. O'Shaughnessy, appeared in Western scientific journals in the 19th century.

In the early 1970s, the anticonvulsant properties of marijuana were again explored, this time through studies on animals. Despite the potential indicated in these studies, the therapeutic benefits of marijuana have been ignored by modern medicine for the last 25 years. In that time, there have been no controlled studies of marijuana in the treatment of human epilepsy. Thus, the body of existing knowledge on this subject rests entirely on informal studies or surveys and is therefore anecdotal.

One of the most frequently cited of these informal studies involves a 24-year-old man who was treated for eight years at a neurology outpatient clinic. He experienced incomplete control of his seizures on a regime of the anticonvulsant drugs, phenobarbitone and phenytoin (Epantin or Pentran), and complained of grand mal seizure attacks as often as every two months. At the age of 22, he began smoking two to five marijuana cigarettes a day, in conjunction with his regular anticonvulsant medication. At this point, his doctors observed that his epileptic seizures completely stopped (Consroe, 1975).

There is some contradictory data about marijuana having both convulsive and anticonvulsive effects. In a few cases, patients have reported experiencing seizures after taking extremely high doses of oral THC. High doses of THC alone have been found to trigger convulsions in animal studies. It is for this reason that Marinol is not thought to be safe or effective for controlling epilepsy.

Researchers believe that another compound found in marijuana, cannabidiol, may have powerful anticonvulsant properties and may counteract the effects of THC. However, small studies in which cannabidiol alone was administered did not yield consistently favourable results. This may point to the fact that the safest and most effective way to treat epilepsy with marijuana is to use all of its compounds together by smoking the plant rather than ingesting its separate ingredients.

If you use marijuana or some other drug to control your epilepsy, be aware that withdrawal from any medication that controls seizures may leave you more susceptible to the seizures. Marijuana is no exception. Whether you are using marijuana alone, or in conjunction with other drugs, you should avoid any drastic change or disruption in the schedule of your medication. If you change too suddenly, you may be more likely to experience seizures. In addition, patients with epilepsy are advised to exercise a great deal of caution when using oral THC. There is not sufficient knowledge about the convulsive or anticonvulsive properties of the single compounds in marijuana to give patients reliable advice. More scientific investigation is necessary.

Today many patients, doctors and healthcare advocates recognize the medical value of marijuana. They are beginning to challenge the stigma surrounding this illegal drug and are demanding to know the truth. With further research, a more thorough understanding of how marijuana can aid in the treatment of epilepsy may be within our reach. In the meantime, many patients with epilepsy are discovering on their own that marijuana can control their seizures. If you are considering using marijuana to control your epilepsy, it is important that you seek the advice of your doctor, as well as other knowledgeable sources. That may be the only way to find out how best to use it in your particular medical situation.

Chapter 10
Pain Management

There are records of marijuana being used as an analgesic, a drug to relieve pain, from ancient China, India, Greece and Rome. Arabic texts referred to marijuana being used to relieve pain as far back as the 2nd century AD. In earlier chapters in this book, we described how patients with cancer, AIDS and various spinal cord and nerve injuries use marijuana to deal with their pain. In later chapters, we will discuss its use for arthritis, migraine and other specific pain problems. Here, in this chapter, we will give you an overview of marijuana to manage pain and cover more of the general pain problems for which marijuana might be helpful.

During the 19th and early 20th centuries, marijuana was a common analgesic in the UK and the United States. It was used less frequently following the development of opiate drugs, or narcotic drugs made from the opium poppy. (For clarification, medical scientists consider 'narcotic' to be synonymous with 'opiate', while botanists and others sometimes use narcotic to refer to any plant with psychoactive properties.) Marijuana does not dissolve in water and therefore injectable preparations are not practical. Opiates do dissolve in water and can be administered by injection, which makes them more reliable in relieving severe pain. Today, severe pain is routinely treated with injectable opiates, including morphine or meperidine (Demerol or Pethidine) and oral derivatives such as codeine, hydrocodone or oxycodone. There are even skin patches of fentanyl (Durogesic) and rectal suppositories of morphine. It's ironic that opiates formed the basis of the antidrug laws drawn up at the Geneva Conference in 1925, and are now widely and extensively used in medicine. Cannabis, which was included almost as an afterthought, when the Egyptian and Turkish delegates claimed it caused lunacy, is still almost entirely absent from the pharmacopoeia in the West.

Opiates can cause physical and psychological dependence (addiction), and most patients who use them report that they are left feeling groggy and unable to focus or think clearly. Opiates can cause severe constipation (tincture of opium is used to treat diarrhoea). They frequently cause nausea, vomiting, dizziness, hallucinations and allergic reactions with flushing, itching and hives. When an individual has side-effects from one opiate, they usually will have similar side-effects with all of the opiates.

There are drugs other than opiates that are commonly prescribed for pain management and do not produce dependence. However, these drugs are often not powerful enough to relieve severe pain. They are synthetic analgesic drugs like paracetamol, Alvedon, Disprol, Panadol, etc. and nonsteroidal (noncortisone) anti-inflammatory drugs (NSAIDs), like aspirin, ibuprofen and many others. When taken daily over long periods of time, aspirin and other NSAIDs can cause stomach ulcers and bleeding tendencies. Many times, one cannot use NSAIDs at all because they 'thin' the blood by affecting the platelet cell in the blood (this is why aspirin is used routinely to prevent heart attacks). If one has a bleeding tendency because of an underlying illness, cancer chemotherapy or a need to take a 'blood thinner' such as warfarin (Marevan), a doctor is very reluctant to use any NSAID because of additional risks of bleeding. Although paracetamol does not 'thin' the blood, large doses can cause fatal liver damage, especially in those who drink alcohol. Long-term use of paracetamol or NSAIDs may also cause kidney failure and a future on a kidney dialysis machine.

Keep in mind that the opiates, NSAIDs and paracetamol are often associated with accidental deaths from overdose. Marijuana cannot kill anyone from overdose, does not cause constipation, nausea, vomiting or stomach ulcers, and actually stimulates one's appetite. As you can see, doctors and patients still need safer, better-tolerated and more effective analgesics.

Despite this obvious shortage of 'patient-friendly' analgesics, modern medicine has given little attention to marijuana as a pain reliever. Medical texts and journals contain only limited information about marijuana as an alternative analgesic. Modern human research studies on the subject did not occur until the 1970s. In one study at the University of Iowa in 1975, hospitalized cancer patients in extreme pain were given low doses of oral THC (Marinol). It provided significant pain relief for up to several hours, and with fewer side-effects than the common analgesic drugs (Mechoulam, 1975; 114). In other tests conducted by the same researchers, inexperienced users found that the psychoactive effects of THC produced anxiety and interfered with its analgesic qualities. However, once patients had become familiar with the psychological high produced by THC, the anxiety resolved and its pain-relieving capacity was fully appreciated.

Modern research has confirmed that THC and other cannabinoids have significant analgesic properties, and do not produce significant physical or psychological dependence compared with opiates. In 1992, scientists discovered nerve receptors in the brain and central nervous system that control the pain caused by nerve damage in the body, or neuropathic pain. These receptors are triggered by a substance that occurs naturally in the body called anandamide. The molecular structure of anandamide is similar to the structure of the cannabinoids found in marijuana. As a result, it is believed that marijuana can trigger these receptors, which would explain its capacity to relieve pain, especially neuropathic pain.

As we described in Chapter 8, on paraplegia and quadriplegia caused by spinal cord injuries, many disabled veterans use marijuana to treat pain from nerve damage caused by their war injuries. They report that none of the nonaddictive medicines give them as much relief as marijuana. In addition, veterans and other amputees who have lost limbs have found that marijuana eases the so-called phantom pain they experience. This pain comes from nerves in the brain that previously communicated with the amputated body part.

More recent studies by research groups at the University of Naples in Italy, the University of California in San Francisco, the University of Michigan and Brown University have shown that cannabinoids found in marijuana, including THC, have a direct effect on pain signals in peripheral tissues of the body, as well as the central nervous system. This means that cannabinoids are also useful in treating local wounds to the flesh or to the skin. This opens up new possibilities for compounds found in marijuana to be used as local anaesthetics.

A growing number of people who live with chronic pain use marijuana because they find it is an effective pain reliever and does not incapacitate or impair their mental functioning in the same way that opiates do. The following is an account of one patient's experience with chronic pain. It began with an occupational injury to the nerves in both of her arms in 1995. She now resides in the state of Massachusetts in the US, but prefers to remain anonymous. She began using marijuana nearly a year after sustaining her injury. The prescription drugs she took before using marijuana did more to disrupt her life and drive her into depression than they did to relieve her pain.

Three years ago, I suffered an injury that ended my 12-year career in electronic engineering. I was working on a metal detection unit, building and testing the product for quality control. On and off for nearly a year, I did heavy repetitive assembly, boring into plastic. Eventually, I began to feel my left hand going numb, and my arm would occasionally fall out on me.

When I first began to notice these problems, I requested electric tools that would spare me some of the physical strain, but instead my company cut back on my labor. I continued working the same way, though less frequently.

The doctor I saw told me I had carpal tunnel syndrome, and he gave me three months of physical therapy. But I knew something was permanently wrong with me months later, when my 6-year-old daughter broke away from my grip as we were walking across a busy street. She was almost hit by a car driving about 40 miles (64 km) per hour.

When I went back to see the doctor, I was given a cortisone steroid shot in my left wrist, and a bottle of codeine pills. I discovered that I couldn't take the pills when I was taking care of my daughter because they knocked me out for hours. We lived on a two-acre mini-farm in Tennessee that I soon found I could not keep. I was either too heavily drugged on the pills, or the pain prevented me from using my hands for anything.

Sometimes the pain felt like electric shocks that began in my elbows, and then shot up through my shoulders and my neck. It got so severe that I ended up wearing hand and wrist splints to avoid further strain. My doctors insisted that this pain in my elbows and my neck was related to the carpal tunnel. They said there wasn't anything that could be done to relieve my pain other than surgery.

It would take 13 months for Workmen's Compensation to authorize the surgery I needed. During that time, I stopped taking the pain relievers because they prevented me from living normally. Having a young daughter required me to be awake and alert, but these drugs made me dizzy and light-headed, and they debilitated me.

For a while, I had a friend who would come over to my house to help me take care of certain things. I couldn't wash my daughter, and I couldn't brush my own hair. During one of her visits, she told me that she thought I should try marijuana. She talked about some of the ways she had heard it was being used by people who had injuries or were ill. It didn't take much to persuade me. I had tried marijuana before, recreationally, and it had never made me feel the way my medicines did.

I soon found that marijuana allowed me to relax without being sedated. It alleviated my pain yet allowed me to focus on other things. I think marijuana also helped to lift me out of the depression I was sinking into. I had gone from being a very active and productive person, and been reduced to a nonfunctional state of mere existence. It was so exasperating for me that I would often just sit down and cry.

I never would have thought that I'd be using marijuana for medical reasons, but then I never would have predicted that my life would take the turn that it did, either. The injury ruined my life as it had been. I lost my ability to work, and my daughter and I eventually lost our home, our animals, and our farm.

When I finally underwent the bilateral carpal tunnel surgery, they found that I had suffered damage to the nerves in my elbows – the ulnar nerves that go from my hands all the way up to my neck. After my surgery, I was again put on narcotics. They gave me Demerol (Pethidine) for nearly a week. The way I felt frightened me so much. I thought my life was going to go foggy and down the drain again, so I stopped, and I went back to using marijuana.

> Marijuana provided a way of getting through the constant pain, and it allowed me to care for everything I had left in my life, like my daughter. I've seen people's lives change as a result of the drugs they've had to take to treat their pain. They can numb you, take away your everyday abilities, and hinder your relationships to family and friends. I've never seen marijuana devastate people who use it medically in this way.
>
> I smoke about a third, or a half of a marijuana cigarette every four hours. That works better than anything else ever has. I still feel the pain coming on sometimes. Nothing could entirely alleviate it, other than removing my nerves. But, it can be lifted when I smoke marijuana, and I can be distracted without losing my ability to function mentally, as a whole person.
>
> In my condition, this is the most I can expect. But I am grateful for it, because I appreciate everything in a different way now. I know my medicine is not legal, but I will never go back to trying to live my life as a zombie. I've already had too much taken away from me. I won't let go of the quality of my life, or the relief I get with this medicine.

Medical scientists do not fully understand how marijuana works as an analgesic. Recent research has revealed that a class of chemicals found in marijuana, called cannabinoids, is very similar to a naturally occurring chemical in the body called anandamide. Numerous nerve receptors throughout the brain and body are triggered by the presence of anandamide. The nerves affected by these receptor firings are involved in pain control, memory and cognition, motor functioning, nausea and vomiting, and internal eye pressure. The discovery of these receptor sites and of the chemical similarities between cannabinoids and anandamide has provoked some new interest in research on the analgesic and other medicinal properties of marijuana.

Whatever the underlying cause, marijuana can be effective in managing pain, but there are certain limitations. First, it may not work for everyone. Second, the accompanying psychological high may be unpleasant for inexperienced users. Third, it appears that marijuana works well for certain kinds of pain but not well for others. In particular, nerve pain seems to be more effectively controlled by marijuana than by commonly prescribed analgesics. While we do not know the specific biological mechanism responsible for the effectiveness of marijuana, we do know that it works differently than opiates and nonsteroidal anti-inflammatory drugs. Better knowledge of this mechanism might one day allow us to develop a more effective treatment for the chronic pain suffered daily by thousands of patients.

Patients who smoke marijuana for pain management get an added benefit. They are able to more precisely control the dose they take into their bodies. The active ingredients in marijuana reach the brain and other sites in the body almost instantaneously when inhaled into the lungs (as opposed to swallowed in pill form or in food). Because of the rapid action of inhaled marijuana, patients can continue smoking until they achieve the desired effect and stop before the psychological high gets more intense than they wish.

While THC (Marinol) has been proven to be effective in some pain management situations, its unwanted psychological side-effects can be too much even for experienced marijuana users. In addition, Marinol is not approved by the US Food and Drug Administration for treatment of any type of pain. It is only approved for prevention of nausea and vomiting in people receiving cancer chemotherapy and for stimulation of appetite in people with AIDS. Any other use (such as for pain) puts the doctor at risk of losing his or her Drug Enforcement Administration (DEA) prescription licence. If a doctor loses his or her DEA licence, it functionally ends the doctor's clinical practice of medicine in the United States. In the UK, doctors are given more freedom to prescribe, but they must take full responsibility for their actions. Marinol is not available in the UK, but another cannabinoid, Nabilone, marketed under the name Cesamet, is. Studies show that while its main action is anti-emetic, it may help in the relief of chronic pain. In 1999, two UK studies will examine the effects of THC (as in Marinol), other cannabinoids (such as Nabilone) and the whole plant on pain management among other things.

Treatment of individuals with persistent (chronic) pain is extremely difficult and risky for doctors. Doctors are warned to avoid prescribing legal narcotics because they may be diverted to the illegal market. The 'War on Drugs' has pushed the prescription of pain medicine away from being a private pact between doctor and patient to being a moral, political and law enforcement issue. In the US, doctors who have placed compassionate care above politics are often investigated and disciplined by state medical boards and the DEA. Sometimes they have restrictions placed on their medical licence and are even sent to 'reeducation conferences' where it is argued that there is no such thing as chronic pain. Although the situation is slightly easier in the UK, the prescribing doctor must still be able to account for his choice of medicine, and take full responsibility for any outcome of its use. That puts enormous pressure on doctors in the UK.

Other drugs that doctors use to help those with chronic pain include antidepressant medications (such as Prozac), antianxiety medications (such as diazepam), and other miscellaneous agents (such as major tranquillizers and drugs commonly used for epilepsy). Many doctors are adamant that marijuana should be added to the list of drugs used to manage pain.

Because doctors often know less about marijuana than patients do, they should be open to all of its potential uses. For example, prior to marijuana prohibition, many women (including Queen Victoria) used marijuana for severe menstrual cramps and today many modern women are rediscovering this fact. The number of painful problems that may respond to marijuana is potentially without limit. It should be understood as one more option in pain management. The patient and doctor should discuss all of the available options and work as a team to make a choice based on the requirements of the individual in pain. If your doctor refuses to work with you on pain management issues, seek another opinion.

Chapter 11
Migraine Headaches

In 1888, Dr W. R. Gowers described migraine headache as 'an affliction characterized by paroxysmal (sudden onset) nervous disturbance, of which headache is the most constant element. The pain is seldom absent and may exist alone, but it is commonly accompanied by nausea and vomiting, and it is often preceded by some sensory disturbance, especially some disorder of the sense of sight. The symptoms are frequently one-sided, and from this character of the headache the name is derived' (Gowers, 1893; 836).

Modern scientists cannot improve upon this accurate observation and description made more than a century ago. Migraine symptoms can last from hours to days. Symptoms usually first appear when one is young and persist until middle age, at which time they may subside or change. The cause is unclear and is related to a complex interaction of blood vessel, nerve tissue and chemical disturbances in the body. Stress, fatigue, menstrual cycles or certain foods may precipitate the headaches.

During the time the description by Dr Gowers was written, physicians were routinely describing marijuana for migraine. In 1891, Dr J. B. Mattison wrote about marijuana and its uses as a pain medication. But in his opinion, the most important use was for migraine (Mattison, 1891). Dr William Osler is one of the most important figures in American medicine and wrote a textbook that, with updated revisions, remains in use today. In

1913, he wrote that marijuana was 'probably the most satisfactory remedy' for migraine (Osler, 1913; 1089).

A small number of patients with migraines have recently 'rediscovered' that marijuana may help alleviate their symptoms. One of the important body chemicals playing a role in migraines is a hormone called serotonin. Some research has shown that THC, one of the active ingredients in marijuana, has an effect on the release of serotonin (Grinspoon, 1997; 126). New drugs developed to treat migraines also work by influencing serotonin. The latest of these is Imigran (sumatriptan), which can be administered orally or by injection and has improved the lives of many people with migraines. When taken orally, many patients find that Imigran is not as effective as they would like. When injected, patients often report that Imigran causes anxiety and chest pains that they find alarming.

Many drugs have been prescribed to treat the pain of severe migraine headaches, including narcotic opiates (drugs made from the opium poppy). Opiates, including injectable morphine and meperidine (Pethidine), as well as oral agents such as codeine, hydrocodone and oxycodone, can cause many side-effects including nausea, vomiting, constipation, drowsiness and mental disturbances including hallucinations. Other drugs such as propranolol (Inderal) and antidepressant drugs such as amitriptyline (Elavil) or fluoxitene (Prozac) are used to decrease the frequency of attacks.

Some people with migraines find that they can use marijuana immediately at the onset of the attack to minimize the severity of the headache. This ability to achieve immediate relief has contributed to an improved quality of life for those who respond to this newly rediscovered 'old' treatment.

Denise Summers is one such patient. At the age of 23, she experienced her first migraine attack while at work. Frightened, dizzy and unable to see out of her right eye, she was taken to a hospital emergency room and given an injection of Imigran. Her symptoms stopped in minutes, but she experienced problems with her ability to talk and think. Within four hours, the pain returned and was just as intolerable as it had been before the injection. At the suggestion of her fiancé, she tried marijuana. Denise has since been medicating regularly with marijuana. She can now eliminate her occasional migraine attacks at the onset of her symptoms, and without any unwanted side-effects.

> I was at work one day pulling patient charts. Suddenly, when I sat up, I felt dizzy, and I saw little white stars in my vision. A coworker saw me trying to keep my balance. When I told her what had just happened, she told me that I should sit down. I sat down, I shut my eyes, and I put my hands over them. Then I laid my head down on the desk. After a few minutes, I stood up and opened my eyes and everything was blurry. I could only see the outline of the person who was standing right in front of me.
>
> Then it started getting worse and I panicked. I thought I was going to go blind. I don't know if it was because I panicked, or what, but I began feeling rather hot and I started to sweat. My coworker noticed that my sleeve was actually wet with perspiration. Then, suddenly, it felt as if someone was driving a screwdriver through my left temple, and the only way I could see anything in focus was if I covered my right eye. Voices were beginning to echo.
>
> I wanted to go lie down and let it pass, but my coworker argued with me. She said I could be having an aneurysm and that I should go to the hospital. So I called the hospital and talked to an emergency room nurse. She told me that I needed to come in as soon as I possibly could. I started to get scared

because I could see everyone else around me was getting scared.

As soon as I got to the emergency room, two nurses immediately began checking my vital signs. They took my temperature, checked my blood pressure, and they were looking into my eyes with a little light. I sat there in a dark examining room for a half-hour, and they came in every five minutes or so to check my vital signs again.

After half an hour, a doctor came in and told me it appeared I was having a migraine. He then told me that he was going to give me a shot of an antimigraine drug that was fairly new, so I would have to remain there under observation for a little while. He gave me a shot of something called Imigran and then he left the room.

At this point, I could see much better, but after receiving the shot, my headache began to spread from my left temple to the whole crown of my head. By the time they came in to check my vital signs again, though, my headache was entirely gone.

When I left the hospital it was about 1:30 PM, and I was extremely drowsy and numb. I couldn't hold a single thought in my head, and I found that I kept thinking about thinking. When my fiancé and my best friend picked me up, my mind was fogged and my speech was slowed. I was incoherent and I couldn't explain to them what had happened to me.

When I got home, I went right to sleep until I woke up at around 5:30 PM. To my dismay, the pain had returned and was just as strong as it had been before. I had been given a prescription for Imigran pills, but it was too late to go to the pharmacy to get it filled. I began to worry about how I was going to feel again.

My fiancé then suggested that I try smoking some marijuana. At first it didn't seem like such a good idea because

I didn't want to do anything that might make my headache worse. But then I remembered what had happened after I had oral surgery nearly a year before. I discovered that a few hits of marijuana worked to take away the pain, much better than the hydrocone they had given me. When I had taken just one hydrocone pill, I nearly passed out, and I started to experience twitching in my vision.

So I decided I'd try the marijuana. I coughed a little after I took the first hit, and when I did, I realized that my head didn't hurt. This is difficult to describe, but my head had been hurting in such a way that any sudden movement, such as laughing or coughing, reverberated in my head, amplifying the pain. I couldn't believe it. I took another hit and I started to relax. Within a few minutes, the pain was completely gone.

After that, I would occasionally get little cluster headaches around my right eye socket. But I found that if I smoked a few hits of marijuana, they would subside. I have not had another attack since I started using marijuana almost a year ago. I never even went in to fill my prescription of Imigran, and I don't think I will ever have to.

Most people who use marijuana for migraines say inhaled marijuana is preferable to oral THC (Marinol) and another cannabinoid, synthetically produced as Nabilone, or to marijuana in foods. This is probably due to the fact that smoking allows patients to immediately achieve the dose they need and then stop. When marijuana is introduced into the body through the digestive system, it takes almost an hour to reach the bloodstream and have an effect. As a result, patients have no way to control their dose because they have to wait so long to feel the effects of the marijuana they have swallowed. This is especially important in the treatment of migraines because symptoms rapidly escalate after the onset and become more difficult to treat.

If you decide to use marijuana to treat your migraine headaches, you will want to experiment with dosage and route of administration to achieve the method that is most effective for you. Then share this information with your doctor. Should you decide to smoke the marijuana, it may be wise to carry a marijuana cigarette with you and discreetly smoke it as soon as you feel the onset of symptoms.

Chapter 12
Arthritis

Arthritis is inflammation of joints and is one of many rheumatic conditions (rheumatism). These are disorders of the body's connective tissue, which is the supporting framework of the body. Arthritis involves the inflammation and degeneration of the cartilage and bone that make up the joint. It can also affect surrounding muscles, tendons and nerves. People with arthritis commonly suffer severe chronic pain and often lose ability to freely move their joints. Since normal functioning joints in the limbs are usually necessary for activities of daily living and employment, arthritis may cause severe disability.

Osteoarthritis is the most common form of arthritis that affects adults. It is characterized by a gradual degeneration of the cartilage in the joints. The many causes of osteoarthritis may range from gradual deterioration, due to normal daily activities, to complications due to sudden trauma to the joints, such as a fracture in the joint surface. Arthritis may also be an autoimmune disorder, that is, a disorder in which the body's immune system attacks some of its own tissues or cells. A common type of autoimmune arthritis that can be very disabling is rheumatoid arthritis.

People with painful rheumatoid conditions are usually treated with common pain relievers (analgesics) like paracetamol (Panadol, Disprin, etc.) or nonsteroidal (noncortisone) anti-inflammatory drugs (NSAIDs) like aspirin, ibuprofen or naproxen. Many patients find that paracetamol or NSAIDs do not sufficiently relieve their pain. Patients with extremely painful rheumatism are sometimes prescribed opiate narcotic drugs (drugs made from the opium poppy).

Aspirin and other NSAIDs have been known to cause stomach ulcers and bleeding when taken daily over long periods of time. Doctors are often reluctant to prescribe NSAIDs to patients because they thin the blood by altering platelet cells. Patients who have a bleeding tendency due to an underlying illness, cancer chemotherapy or a need to take a blood thinner such as warfarin (Marevan) run a heightened risk of bleeding due to NSAIDs. While paracetamol does not thin the blood, high doses can cause fatal liver damage. Long-term use of paracetamol or NSAIDs may also cause kidney failure and the need for ongoing kidney dialysis.

Opiates can cause physical and psychological dependence, and most patients who use them complain about feeling groggy and being unable to focus or think clearly. Opiates also can cause severe constipation (tincture of opium is used to treat diarrhoea). They frequently cause nausea, vomiting, dizziness, hallucinations and allergic reactions with flushing, itching and hives. When an individual has side-effects from one opiate, they usually will have similar side-effects with all of the opiates.

Keep in mind that NSAIDs, paracetamol and opiates are often associated with accidental deaths from overdose. With marijuana there is no danger from overdose, and marijuana does not cause constipation, nausea, vomiting or stomach ulcers, and actually stimulates one's appetite. Doctors and patients still need safer, better-tolerated and more effective analgesics.

Many patients with rheumatism are now using marijuana, which has long been known to have anti-inflammatory properties (Formukong, 1988). In 1997, at an annual meeting of the US Society for Neuroscience in New Orleans, Dr Kenneth Hargreaves of the University of Texas reported that synthetic cannabinoids can relieve the inflammation associated with arthritis when injected directly at the site of injury. This finding supports patients' claims that some of the consequences of inflammation, such as impaired mobility, are improved by marijuana.

Many arthritis patients say they use marijuana to relieve chronic pain. If you are considering using it for this purpose, you may want to read Chapter 10, on pain management, after completing this chapter.

Theresa Escue, who lives in Florida, is one of an increasing number of people with rheumatism who use marijuana to control pain and inflammation. Though she was thought to have received only minor injuries and strains following a 1975 car accident in Dallas, Texas, her doctors believe that the arthritis she developed years later may have been exacerbated by her injuries.

> Marijuana was something I never felt any benefit from until I was in a car accident in 1975. It occurred right in front of the apartment building I lived in, and I waited in shock with the building manager for an ambulance to arrive. I was in extreme pain and I couldn't move. All I remember is that he gave me a marijuana joint, and he told me that it would help me until the ambulance came. Miraculously, it did. It made me relax, and it lessened the pain I was feeling all throughout my body.
>
> I had tried marijuana once before my accident. It made me fall asleep, so I never wanted to do it again. In fact, although it made me feel better immediately after the accident, I didn't use it again, until my arthritis set in nearly ten years later.
>
> Since the accident, I had felt some pain in places in my

arms, my shoulders, and my back. But, I never paid much attention, until it got so severe that getting out of bed became difficult for me. I eventually had to get rid of my waterbed because I couldn't easily get out of it.

When I finally went to see a doctor, I was told I had rheumatoid arthritis, and that it was likely triggered by the accident I'd had years earlier. Two of the drugs they gave me were naproxen and Lodine (both are NSAIDs). One problem I had with these drugs was that, after a while, their effectiveness would wear off. I had to switch what I was taking, or I found that I had to take greater amounts.

Though I never had any real problems with side-effects, the more I had to take for the drugs to work, the more I felt like they were having a negative effect on my body. They were slowly dulling me, and the thought of continuing that way was depressing. I've never known if this was a consequence of the medications or not, but I was often in a state of anxiety while taking them. The anxiety would make me tense, and the tension would exacerbate my arthritis.

But the biggest problem for me was the cost. These medications cost me a few hundred dollars a month. Depending on how much I was taking, or how frequently, it was simply more than I could afford. For this reason, mainly, last year I quit taking them altogether and I began using marijuana regularly. The difference in the way I feel with marijuana is that it makes me more relaxed. I don't have the anxiety that causes tension anymore. My flare-ups don't stay with me long enough to make me feel debilitated.

My pain usually begins to set in at the end of the day. It can range from a dull ache to a stabbing pain in a joint. My shoulder blades become so tight that I can't sit, and I can't stand up. Nothing helps unless I can relax. Marijuana helps me to relax and it steadily eases my pain. The effect doesn't wear off, and I only have to take a couple hits. I can just take the amount I need.

The only problem with marijuana is the stigmatism and the stress that it can cause. But until there is a better way for me to live the rest of my life with my condition, I will continue to use it because it works.

Arthritis commonly affects mature adults. Many of them reluctantly accept it as a more or less unavoidable consequence of ageing. Given that the drugs usually prescribed often lead to unwanted side-effects, and are expensive or ineffective, it is not surprising that many patients with arthritis turn to marijuana as an alternative. Those who grew up during the 1960s and 1970s are quite likely to have been exposed to marijuana use when it became associated with youthful rebellion. Senior citizens are less likely to have had prior experience with marijuana. Many seniors with arthritis might benefit from marijuana, but are reluctant to try it because of their unfamiliarity with and subsequent fear of marijuana.

In an interesting historical sidelight, the political campaign that led to the 1996 passage of Proposition 215 in California, which permits medical patients to use marijuana under state law, got under way because of arthritis. Anna Boyce, a semi-retired registered nurse living in Orange County, was a volunteer serving on a neighbourhood watch patrol. One day, she discovered a local home that had been burglarized and called the sheriff's deputies. They searched the home, which belonged to a prominent local attorney, and in the process discovered a small amount of marijuana. The burglars were never caught, but the attorney, who had been using the marijuana to control his rheumatoid arthritis, was arrested and charged with possession of a controlled substance.

Anna Boyce was so outraged by the consequences that she

launched a campaign to permit patients to use marijuana as medicine. Eventually, she succeeded in getting a bill to that effect introduced in the California Legislature. On two occasions, in 1994 and 1995, this bill passed both houses with bipartisan support only to be vetoed by Governor Pete Wilson. In 1996, following a massive petition drive, the vetoed bill became a state initiative and was put on the ballot as Proposition 215. California voters passed Proposition 215 by a 56 per cent to 44 per cent margin.

Chapter 13
Asthma

Asthma is a breathing disorder caused by the inflammation and swelling of the small airways (bronchioles) inside the lungs. When the bronchioles become inflamed, swollen and filled with mucus, the airways become narrow and make it difficult to breathe. Symptoms of asthma attacks may include breathlessness, wheezing, mucus production and/or coughing. Asthma symptoms may be triggered by allergies (such as pollen, house dust, animal dander, etc.), respiratory infections (viral or bacterial), air pollutants and exercising in cold, dry air. Anyone of any age can develop asthma. In the UK, there are more than 3 million asthmatics, and every week around 40 people die from asthma in this country.

Asthma attacks are typically treated with 'bronchodilators', drugs that work by relaxing and opening the bronchioles. Bronchodilators can be taken in pill form, or they can be delivered by inhalation or by injection. There are many different types of bronchodilators. Many produce undesirable side-effects of some sort. Among these are dizziness, restlessness, insomnia, muscle twitching with shakiness, nausea, vomiting and seizures. In rare circumstances, bronchodilators have been associated with cardiac arrest in people with asthma.

Not all 'asthma inhalers' are in the bronchodilator category. Some inhalers work by reducing inflammation (anti-inflammatories) and some work by blocking a nerve called the vagus nerve. The medical trend over recent decades has been to embrace inhalation-type treatments in asthma to try to minimize the side-effects of the oral or injectable drugs.

Cortisone-type steroids are often used to treat asthma. They are given to reduce the inflammation or swelling of the bronchioles. Doctors try to limit the use of oral or injectable cortisone to short periods of time, because over long periods of time it can cause serious side-effects. As mentioned in previous chapters, some of the potential long-term side-effects are softening and loss of bone (osteoporosis), susceptibility to infection (because of negative effects on the immune system), cataracts, stomach ulcers and seizures. When people with asthma need cortisone-type steroids over a long period of time, doctors prefer an inhalation method, but when the asthma is very severe, regular use of risky oral cortisone-type steroids may be life-saving. As with other medical therapy, you and your doctor must discuss the benefits versus the risks.

While at first it may seem ridiculous to treat asthma by smoking marijuana, Muslims in Arabia and Indonesia have done it for centuries. British physicians witnessed its use for spasmodic asthma attacks in India in the 19th century. In the US, marijuana was reported as an effective treatment for asthma as early as 1910. Modern studies have confirmed that THC, the psychoactive compound in marijuana, is an effective bronchodilator. In one 1974 study, both smoked and oral THC were found to increase the bronchial diameter for a period of more than two hours. When compared to isoproterenol (Isuprel), a standard bronchodilator, smoked marijuana was slightly less effective but lasted longer (Mechoulam, 1986; 149).

Today, a growing number of people who suffer with asthma are using marijuana, as an addition to or a replacement for their standard treatments. For many, marijuana works as well as their pharmaceutical drugs, without the unwanted side-effects. Others insist that marijuana works better.

The asthmatic symptoms that Florida resident Kim Morgan experienced as a child diminished as soon as she reached puberty. At 23, however, Kim's asthma returned. She medicated regularly with standard drugs. By the age of 30, she had grown weary of the side-effects and the cost, and she was concerned about her overall health.

A friend prompted her to try marijuana recreationally. That's when she discovered it was possible to treat her asthma without relying on the unwanted pharmaceuticals.

> In 1987, I was diagnosed with adult onset asthma. I had been working an 11:00 PM to 7:00 AM shift at a manufacturing plant. The fall season was hitting as it normally does in Florida. I left the plant one morning and it seemed as if the weather had changed overnight. I think that's what brought it on. By the time I got to my car, I couldn't breathe. I began wheezing and turning blue. It felt as if a huge fist had grabbed both my lungs and squeezed.
>
> I stayed in the hospital for two days. They gave me a shot of epinephrine (adrenaline), and it helped me breathe. Then they ran a series of tests on me, and gave me my diagnosis. I left the hospital with a fistful of prescriptions.
>
> One of the things I took was called theophylline (aminophylline). It's supposed to relax the smooth muscle in your lungs so oxygen can get through. This drug has been credited with putting thousands of patients in hospital emergency rooms every year. When I took it, it made me shake in my hands and my extremities, and it badly upset my stomach. At first, they started me out at a low dosage, but then my body built up a tolerance, so they had to increase it. I went from 150 mg to 1200 mg over the seven years that I took it.
>
> I also used a couple of different inhalers. Some of them helped if I had a sudden attack. The others were steroids of

which I had to keep a certain amount in my system. I didn't like the way I felt on these drugs. Often times I could not sleep at night, or I would feel really nervous.

There was a period of about six months during which I was in and out of the hospital. I would wake up in the middle of the night unable to breathe. My doctor wasn't sure if the type or dosage of medicine I was taking was right. Throughout the day, for any reason, I would have an attack. The precursors of an attack start with a sensation in your gut. Then you may have to go to the bathroom. Though an attack usually came on immediately, if I paid attention, I might be able to catch it with my inhaler.

I coped with my asthma for over seven years in this way. At different times, my health was either better or worse. Then, in 1995, I decided I wanted to stop taking these pharmaceuticals. I had turned 30, and I began to feel like I didn't want to put them in my body anymore. At the time, my doctor was about to put me on more steroids, and I had reached a point where I felt I couldn't go along with it anymore.

I had first tried smoking marijuana three years before, and I noticed that I was breathing a lot more easily. I tried it two more times, and I had the same experience each time. But it didn't really occur to me that I could use it as a medicine, until I stopped taking my pharmaceuticals.

When I smoke marijuana, the frequency of my attacks decreases to zero. They go away. I stopped going to my doctor's appointments because they were costing me an arm and a leg. I just canceled my next appointment and I never went back. I thought if I told a doctor what I was doing to treat myself, I was sure to be put in jail.

I've smoked marijuana as many ways as you possibly can. No, I don't feel like smoking has been as detrimental to my lungs as it may be to other people. In fact, I think my overall health is better than anyone else I know. The process of smoking it is similar to how doctors treat asthma conventionally. They use a ventilation process, with a little machine that vaporizes liquid medicine. The medicine goes into an oxygen stream and gets to the same place marijuana goes. This is very site specific. Regardless, there are many methods people can choose from to medicate with marijuana.

I keep an inhaler, the weakest one, for back up, in case I have a dry spell, and I can't smoke marijuana. But it's now almost two years old. If I smoke marijuana regularly, I don't have any problems. I also have an overall lessening of symptoms. I take it daily. I try not to smoke it during the day, but I do at night before I go to bed.

I've never even considered Marinol (synthetic THC). It doesn't contain as many compounds as are in marijuana. These compounds all work together. I think that before we can determine what parts of marijuana produce certain effects, we need more practical research.

I've had people who disapprove tell me I ought to be in jail. That's not a very compassionate way of looking at things. I've tried to explain, but some people don't seem to want to understand. I've always stayed away from the political arena, but I think it's time for me to take a stand in some way. It's not just important for me, but for people who need marijuana to treat more serious illnesses, as well. No, I don't want to be a martyr, and I don't want to go to jail, but I will do what I can to stay healthy, and I will try to make sure others have the same option, too.

If you are considering using marijuana to control asthma, keep in mind that some patients cannot tolerate any type of smoke. Because smoke can trigger asthma attacks in some people, you should be very cautious. Marijuana smoke does contain various tars and other impurities and can cause chronic inflammation of the bronchial tree (bronchitis) in heavy smokers.

To avoid the risks of smoking, marijuana can be taken orally in the form of THC pills, or it can be cooked into foods and eaten. Either way, the active ingredients are absorbed very slowly, so this will never be a way to get quick relief. On the other hand, it can be a way to permanently maintain a minimal level of marijuana in your system in order to prevent attacks. Some researchers have experimented with administering THC through a spray inhaler and have got good results. Unfortunately, recent studies have also shown that THC droplets can irritate the lungs, so spray inhalers are not yet a good alternative.

One possible way of eliminating marijuana smoke irritation is through the process of vaporization. The unique compounds in marijuana (cannabinoids) vaporize around 190 degrees centigrade, but the plant skeleton burns, releasing smoke, around 560 degrees centigrade. If the temperature of the vaporizer is held to around 190 degrees centigrade, it should be possible to deliver vaporized cannabinoids without some of the irritants contained in smoke (Rosenthal, 1997; 108–109). Unfortunately, there are laws in the United States that prevent the sale of drug paraphernalia. These laws have impeded the development of vaporizer technology. In the Canadian city of Vancouver, British Columbia, 'Hemp BC' sells a model by mail, but they warn purchasers on their website (http://www.hempbc.com) that importing this model may be illegal because of paraphernalia laws. Drug paraphernalia may be sold in the UK, and there are a variety of products available, including vaporizers and 'bongs'.

It is possible that further research will establish better ways to administer THC, or that other compounds in marijuana will prove to be even better in treating asthma. It might one day be possible to create a preparation of marijuana that preserves most of its active ingredients, and which then could be sprayed directly into the lungs. However, developing such a spray would require a higher commitment to medical marijuana research than presently exists. In the meantime, the number of asthmatics treating themselves with marijuana is growing because many find that the available treatments are far less satisfactory and extremely expensive.

Chapter 14
Crohn's Disease and Other Digestive Problems

It is well known that marijuana can treat nausea and vomiting while stimulating appetite in patients with cancer and AIDS. Marijuana may also be beneficial to people with any gastrointestinal (stomach and intestines) problem that includes nausea, vomiting, poor appetite and pain.

Marijuana is used by some patients with irritable bowel syndrome, which is a common, often painful and disabling condition that may be associated with nausea, vomiting, bloating and changes in bowel habits. When people see doctors for abdominal pain, the most common diagnosis is irritable bowel. Irritable bowel syndrome is probably caused by abnormal bowel contractions but there are no ulcers, bleeding or deaths caused by irritable bowel. If you have a diagnosis of irritable bowel syndrome and develop intestinal bleeding, you should revisit your doctor. Unfortunately, bowel cancer and inflammatory bowel disease can still develop in those with irritable bowel. Some people mistakenly assume the bleeding to be from irritable bowel while delaying the diagnosis of a potentially life-threatening illness.

Inflammatory bowel disease is much different from irritable bowel syndrome. Inflammatory bowel disease includes patients with conditions called Crohn's disease (regional enteritis) and ulcerative colitis. A patient with inflammatory bowel disease may get very ill, require many toxic medications, and need extensive life-saving surgery. Doctors do not know the exact cause of irritable bowel syndrome or inflammatory bowel disease and treatment is often unsatisfactory. We are now going to focus on the inflammatory bowel disease called Crohn's disease.

The inflammation from Crohn's disease can cause ulcers, bleeding and scar formation that may lead to intestinal blockage. As a result, patients suffer intestinal cramps and spasms, nausea and vomiting, loss of appetite and weight, severe diarrhoea and rectal bleeding. Many patients suffering with Crohn's disease have recently discovered that marijuana can be useful in treating their symptoms.

Doctors attempt to treat Crohn's disease with anti-inflammatory or immune-suppressing drugs, including cortisone-type steroids such as prednisone. These drugs can produce severe side-effects, including nausea and vomiting, mood swings, depression, sleeplessness, fluid retention with bloating and drastic weight gain. Long-term cortisone can also cause diabetes, cataracts, stomach problems, abnormal blood potassium levels, immune system deficiency, thinning of the bones (osteoporosis), redistribution of body fat (which may change facial appearance), muscle wasting, seizures and countless other problems. In spite of the best modern medical care, Crohn's disease often worsens. Patients may still require surgery to drain an abscess, remove diseased intestine or control bleeding.

Candice Kluge has lived with Crohn's disease since 1994. Two years ago, after taking high levels of cortisone-type steroids, she developed severe osteoporosis, which is thinning of the bones. Candice then suffered a severe seizure as doctors withdrew her medication. Because of this seizure, she sustained a serious back injury and became nearly suicidal. In the following account, Candice describes how she discovered marijuana, how it improved her health, and how she was then able to stop treating her Crohn's disease with potentially dangerous pharmaceuticals.

I am someone who uses marijuana to live with Crohn's disease. I am out of the closet, so to speak, however reluctantly. I'm 42 years old, and I have two children and four grandchildren. My husband just completed school, and he currently works as a computer technician at our local hospital here in Washburn, Wisconsin.

My family has had a difficult time understanding my marijuana use as a medical need. While I have been medicating with marijuana for about a year now, neither of my children, nor my husband, use any drugs whatsoever.

I found out I had Crohn's disease after the summer of my third year in college, as I was struggling to pass a math class. I had entered school in 1991, because I'd injured my right arm and it ruined my career as a welder. I wanted to find another vocation for myself.

On the morning of September 23, I woke up with the most incredible pain in my stomach area. It felt as if my intestines had literally blow up overnight. When I managed to get up and go to the bathroom, I had diarrhea and was losing unbelievable amounts of blood. I was so terrified by what was happening to me that I remember thinking, 'Oh God, no one could live through something like this.'

An hour later, I ended up in the emergency room. They gave me an IV right away, and then they weighed me. I had gone from 130 to 160 pounds (58 to 71 kg), seemingly overnight. Within the first hour, I had a semi-diagnosis, but it was unusual that Crohn's disease would show up at my age, which was 38. After a while, I was firmly diagnosed with Crohn's disease.

I understood nothing about what this meant for a very long time. In fact, I was disappointed by the care I was given after my diagnosis. For months, I went without a doctor explaining anything to me. All I was told was that there was no known cause, and no known cure, for what I had. Meanwhile, I was terrified because I was bleeding from the rectum, and I felt like my stomach was going to blow up.

Because I didn't know anything about the disease, I began to feel responsible, looking back at everything I had done in my life. I tried to figure out what I could have done wrong, to cause such sickness in my body. It wasn't until much later that I found out Crohn's disease can be hereditary. Then I found out that my grandmother's sisters had had it. Men seem to have it more often than women, and symptoms usually occur prior to the age of 20, or after the age of 60.

For a year I took narcotics for the pain and anti-inflammatory drugs to stop the stomach spasms. They just didn't work. I also took steroids, like prednisone, to stun my immune system. I took something called Losec (omeprazole SA), which was supposed to stop ulcer-type symptoms, and it made my hair fall out by the handful. I developed atrophy from one or a combination of these treatments. My muscles were so weak, I just couldn't walk. What was really alarming is how my body blew up due to the steroids. My weight had gone from 130 to 240 pounds (57 to 106 kg).

What was crazy about all of this was that my body was blowing up while I couldn't even eat. The disease had taken away my appetite. No one understood this. My father even accused me of overeating. He thought I was hiding in the closet eating Twinkies. But my main symptom was constant diarrhea. I had to go to the bathroom anywhere from 30 to 50 times per day. Many times, it was so bad that I had to get into the shower and spray myself with water. They gave me everything under the sun to stop the diarrhea, and nothing worked. At one time, I was using such heavy doses of Imodium (loperamide; a drug to treat diarrhea), along with the narcotics, that I ended up with an obstruction in my bowel, and passed an eight-pound stool in the hospital. I nearly underwent surgery to remove it.

I lived like this for about three years. Then, one day, my nephew came to my bedside with a bowl of pot. He was shocked to see how sick I was. By that point, I felt that I had tried everything. I had looked in every direction for a way to treat myself and found nothing. I'd seen an Indian medicine man and a faith healer. I'd contacted the National Organization for Rare Diseases, thinking they might be able to tell me something my doctors couldn't. All I found out was that they classify Crohn's disease as an 'unknown and incurable disease'.

I truly felt like I was dying in a dark bedroom. I had to do something to change the state I was in. There was some tension beginning to affect my marriage, and I was desperate.

The minute I smoked some of the marijuana my nephew had brought me, I felt all of my intestines stand up to attention. It was an actual physical feeling, like everything inside me was pulling together. Within a few minutes, I was up and out of bed making dinner. It had been so long since I'd felt that good, I knew it would help me to continue using marijuana. But after my nephew left, I didn't have easy access to it. I continued with my regular treatments and used marijuana for relief when I could, which was rare. At that time, I also tried getting a prescription for Marinol (oral THC), but wasn't able to.

In 1995, I was hospitalized because I had become so toxic due to the steroids. I didn't really know what was wrong, but I couldn't walk. I was really scared. The doctors kept me in the hospital, and they put me on an IV steroid drip. I had developed steroid-induced osteoporosis and lost 40 per cent of my bone mass. This explained the crushing sensation I'd been feeling in my ribcage and shoulders.

In the process of withdrawing from the steroids, I suffered a grand mal seizure. My doctor was there when it happened, and he just looked on. After the seizure was over, I felt a terrible pain in my back. When I complained to my doctor about the pain, he became extremely annoyed because he would have to treat me 'for that, too'. Following this whole ordeal, I became suicidal. I called a crisis hotline that put me in touch with a psychiatrist. The psychiatrist referred me to a doctor in southern Wisconsin who examined me for my back pain. He found that I had three compression fractures from the T7 to the T10 vertebrae in my spine, as a result of the seizure.

That's when I knew I had to stop taking these pharmaceuticals. They weren't really helping me, and they were causing too many other problems. I had suffered serious damage to my body from taking them, and none of this happened when I used marijuana. It gave me an appetite and allowed me to eat on a regular basis. With Crohn's disease, it's important to eat several small meals a day. Marijuana also stopped my stomach spasms.

When you smoke marijuana, you don't have to smoke much to get an effect. I have built up a tolerance to its psychoactive effect, but it still relieves my symptoms. I use it about every four hours. I suffer if I don't use it. Within twelve hours, I get diarrhea and my intestinal spasms start up again.

For the last six months, I have been able to obtain a steady supply of marijuana that I use to medicate. I have not taken any more steroids or anti-inflammatory drugs since then. The only other things I feel I need to take are some calcium products so that I don't lose more bone.

I am now treated by a family physician in our home-town. The first time I mentioned my marijuana use, she walked out of the room yelling. But because marijuana has worked so well, I've recently got her support and she gave me a recommendation.

My health has changed drastically since one year ago, when I first started medicating with marijuana. I've been able to lose 100 pounds (45 kg) within that time. I've gone from 248 to 150 pounds (110 to 67 kg). My system is back to normal, and I have one normal bowel movement a day. I take about four or five puffs, about four times a day. My sickness also used to affect my sleeping, as I would wake up in pain. I would only get about three hours of sleep every night. Now my day begins at about 5:00 AM and ends at 11:00 PM.

The problem now is that every day I'm afraid I'm going to go to jail. I went to breakfast this morning and I saw two police officers. It made me feel uncomfortable because my medicine makes me a criminal, and it shouldn't be that way. I don't want to live outside the rules of this society, but I can't live the way I was, and I've been given no other choice.

I remember talking to a nurse at Johns Hopkins once. I was trying to explain my marijuana use. She just stopped me and said, 'Oh, we know it works for Crohn's disease.' So many other patients like me know that it works, and so do a lot of our healthcare providers. Why then does it have to be illegal?

The ability of marijuana to reduce nausea and stimulate appetite is of obvious benefit for people with Crohn's disease. Marijuana may also have anti-inflammatory properties. The chronic diarrhoea and bleeding suffered by patients with Crohn's disease occurs in part because of the inflammation of the inside lining of the intestines. Patients who use marijuana to treat treatment may receive the double benefit of its ability to reduce nausea and inflammation. As a result, many such patients are reporting dramatic effects achieved with marijuana, just as Candice Kluge did in the story above.

If you are suffering from any condition that produces nausea and vomiting, such as kidney dialysis, you may benefit from marijuana. Similarly, if you are unable to eat enough food, marijuana may help. Finally, there is a possibility that marijuana relieves symptoms that are caused by inflammation. In all cases, tell your doctor what you are doing and why and how you are using marijuana as medicine. You and your doctor can then work together in a way that will allow you to make a more informed choice based on all of the options that are available.

Chapter 15

Other Reported Uses of Medical Marijuana

The previous chapters of this book have described medical conditions for which large numbers of people have reported some benefit from marijuana. In this chapter, we will cover a wide variety of other conditions for which there are fewer people making such reports. Many of these other conditions are related to those for which there are numerous reports. As a result, there is good reason to believe that they, too, might be helped by marijuana.

Recent discoveries about the medical uses of marijuana have been made more frequently by patients than by doctors and scientists. Our confidence in these discoveries rests in large part on the number of patients, from all walks of life and from all possible locations, who all report essentially the same observations about the capacity of marijuana to relieve a certain set of symptoms. It is hard to imagine that such a wide spectrum of people are all making up the same story or are all deluded in the same way. The previous chapters were all based on such widespread and well-documented claims about marijuana.

However, the fact that fewer patients may be reporting that marijuana is helpful with regard to other diseases and symptoms does not necessarily mean that their claims are any less valid. Rather, it is possible that these patients are among a vanguard learning about new applications for marijuana. Knowledge about its effectiveness has to start somewhere. Nonetheless, until such claims are validated, either by traditional research or by more widespread reporting of the same phenomena, they should be viewed with caution.

Some of the claims we will review in this chapter are more widely reported than others. We have arranged the sections below to reflect that. The earlier sections describe claims about medicinal uses of marijuana for which there is greater reason to be confident than the claims described in later sections. On the other hand, claims about marijuana described in the later sections may be no less valid. Instead, they may simply be part of a new body of knowledge not yet fully developed.

Nausea and Vomiting

It is widely known that the nausea caused by AIDS and cancer chemotherapy can be dramatically reduced by marijuana. It is logical to assume that nausea resulting from other disorders can also be helped by marijuana. This seems to be the case. Patients suffering from kidney failure, with or without dialysis, are often severely affected by nausea. Many of these patients are now discovering that marijuana is the best medicine for reducing their nausea.

There are many other medical conditions that cause intolerable nausea and vomiting. Regardless of the cause, there is a large body of anecdotal evidence (stories told by patients) indicating that marijuana has a unique ability to reduce nausea and vomiting, and may, in fact, be one of the most powerful medicines available for this purpose. In addition to the diseases already discussed, other conditions that produce intolerable nausea and vomiting include severe chronic congestive heart failure, severe diabetes with wasting, liver failure, and a wide variety of stomach and intestinal (gastrointestinal) problems.

Eating Disorders and Appetite Problems

Another medicinal property of marijuana, which is widely accepted, is its ability to stimulate appetite. Patients with AIDS and those being treated with cancer chemotherapy are increasingly aware of this. Some claim that the capacity of marijuana to stimulate appetite has quite literally saved their lives. But there are many other medical conditions that provoke a loss of appetite. It is logical to assume that marijuana would be useful for any of them.

Physical conditions are not the only cause of loss of one's appetite. Anorexia nervosa is an example of a condition in which the loss of appetite can be psychologically induced. Unfortunately, many young women in our society have fallen victim to standards of beauty which unduly emphasize being thin. This has led to a variety of eating disorders of which anorexia nervosa is only one. In situations where psychological treatment has not solved the problem, an appetite stimulant like marijuana might be of use.

Moderate Pain Management

Marijuana can be a very effective pain-reliever (analgesic), not just for severe pain but also for the management of more moderate pain. To many doctors, marijuana represents a new class of pain medicine that can be used as an alternative to conventional drugs. In many situations, paracetamol (Hedex, Disprol, Panadol, etc.), nonsteroidal (noncortisone) anti-inflammatory drugs (NSAIDs), like aspirin and ibuprofen, or even opiate narcotics, are simply not effective. In other situations, these drugs produce a wide variety of unacceptable side-effects. Given its analgesic properties, marijuana should be considered as an alternative. In addition, if a condition is severe enough to warrant the prescription of opiate narcotics, like morphine, then the condition is severe enough to warrant consideration of marijuana. Marijuana is not as psychologically debilitating as morphine, and does not cause significant physical dependence.

The chemicals in marijuana called cannabinoids represent an entirely new class of drugs. This means that those who cannot use conventional drugs because of side-effects may still be able to use marijuana. For example, if someone develops hallucinations, vomiting and constipation with morphine use, the patient will probably have the same side-effects if other opiate narcotics are prescribed. However, since there is no chemical relationship between marijuana and opiate narcotics, marijuana is a viable option for a doctor to suggest to a patient unable to take opiate narcotics.

Because marijuana has anti-inflammatory properties in addition to its pain-relieving capacity, it might be useful in a variety of disorders that leave patients with very painful symptoms. For example, ankylosing spondylitis, a form of arthritis in the back, is a very uncomfortable disorder from which some people have attained relief using marijuana. Patients with spinal stenosis, which is a painful compression of a spinal nerve, have also reported treating themselves successfully with marijuana. In both cases, the relief reported might be due either to the analgesic properties of marijuana or to the anti-inflammatory properties.

There are other gastrointestinal diseases caused by inflammation for which some patients have used marijuana successfully. Examples include colitis, hepatitis, gastritis and pancreatitis.

Spasms and Tremors

The ability of marijuana to control the muscle spasms associated with multiple sclerosis and spinal cord injury is well documented. Some patients are now reporting that marijuana may also be useful in blocking tremors (shakes) caused by diseases of the brain and spinal cord. Nerve pathways from the brain and spinal cord often function to suppress or slow down muscle activity so the muscles can be used in a coordinated fashion. When there is damage to the central nervous system, this 'calming' effect of the higher nerve centres is often destroyed.

Some patients who have suffered strokes and other brain disorders report that marijuana prevents tremors. Tremors common to conditions such as Parkinson's Disease may also respond to marijuana. Dystonias and tics are neurologic conditions associated with abnormal muscle tone and muscle movement. These are seen with disorders such as Tourette's Syndrome, cerebral palsy, drug side-effects and rare inherited diseases. Patients with these conditions may also benefit from marijuana. If such reports are corroborated, it will be of great significance, as the drugs currently being used to treat these diseases are clearly inadequate.

Stroke, Parkinson's Disease, Alzheimer's Disease

In an April 1998 study at the US National Institute for Mental

Health, in Maryland, researchers concluded that cannabinoids found in marijuana may actually protect brain cells against a destructive chemical reaction that occurs during a stroke. This is especially ironic since much of the debate about marijuana has centred around the assumption that it destroys brain cells. During a stroke, the brain releases toxic levels of the neurotransmitter, glutamate, causing irreversible damage to brain cells. Currently, doctors who treat victims of stroke rely on antioxidants, such as vitamins C and E, to protect brain cells by blocking glutamate production.

In this study, A. J. Hampson and his colleagues found that the cannabinoids, THC and CBD, also act as potent antioxidants. In fact, they were more effective than vitamins C and E. Cannabinoids easily pass through the so-called blood-brain barrier that prevents foreign molecules from entering the brain. As a result, researchers have concluded that these compounds hold advantages over other antioxidants, and if given to a stroke victim quickly enough may limit brain damage.

The discovery that cannabinoids can protect healthy brain cells by blocking glutamate release may mean that marijuana might be useful in the treatment of other brain diseases, such as Parkinson's and Alzheimer's. Parkinson's Disease involves the destruction of brain cells that produce dopamine, a neurotransmitter which is essential to the normal functioning of the central nervous system. People with Parkinson's have muscular tremors, impaired motor control, partial facial paralysis and weakness. Alzheimer's Disease also involves damage to brain cells and is associated with progressive memory loss. No studies have yet been done to specifically test the effectiveness of marijuana in the treatment of these two disorders.

Diabetes

Diabetes is a disorder of the body's metabolic, or energy-producing, process. Most commonly, diabetes involves the inability to produce sufficient amounts of the hormone insulin.

One long-term side-effect of diabetes is damage to nerve fibres of the autonomic nervous system which, amongst other things, controls the gastrointestinal tract. It is estimated that about 75 per cent of all diabetics have gastrointestinal symptoms. The most common of these symptoms is diabetic gastroparesis, or paralysis of the stomach. People who have diabetic gastroparesis have trouble digesting food due to the failure of the stomach muscles to contract and relax.

Commonly reported symptoms include bloating, acid build-up, nausea and vomiting, and appetite loss. Since marijuana helps relieve problems of nausea and vomiting, and stimulates appetite, many people who suffer diabetes report using it to relieve their symptoms.

Sleep Disturbances and Stress Reduction

Insomnia is a problem for millions of people. The cause is not well understood. For some, it is a problem of anxiety and mental stress. For others, the cause is more physical and related to accompanying disease. Since a portion of the people who use marijuana complain that it makes them sleepy, others are taking advantage of this property of marijuana and use it to help them attain sleep. If sleepiness is desired because of insomnia, marijuana may be an option. It hardly matters whether it works by reducing anxiety and mental stress or by inducing sleep directly.

Many people use marijuana to reduce stress. Most would

classify themselves as recreational users. They do not recognize that using a drug to reduce stress is no different than a physician prescribing a tranquillizer for the same purpose. Stress is becoming a more serious problem in our fast-paced society. Mounting evidence indicates that it exacerbates a broad spectrum of serious physical disorders. It is hard to argue from a public policy standpoint that an illegal drug like marijuana should be used for a condition like stress. But it is possible to make the argument from a medical standpoint in cases where stress is a serious problem and the existing tranquillizing drugs are either inadequate or cause unwanted side-effects.

Addiction

While the reports are not widespread, there are many individuals who now claim that marijuana use enables them to give up alcohol, heroin or cocaine. It may seem paradoxical to use one drug to help give up another drug. But, given the relatively benign nature of marijuana as compared to all three of these addictive substances, it is clear that the addicted person will be far better off, physically and mentally, using marijuana rather than these more toxic substances. Long-term studies of marijuana use have shown no adverse effects. In addition, many in our society condone the use of methadone, an opiate narcotic, to control heroin addiction. Marijuana is far less harmful.

Mood Disorders

Many are concerned about the negative psychological side-effects of marijuana. As a result, little attention has been given to its possibly therapeutic potential in the treatment of psychological disorders. Some patients have found the mood-altering effects of marijuana to be helpful for treating mood disorders such as anxiety, depression and bipolar (manic-depressive) illness. Using marijuana to treat mood disorders was described in medical writings in the 19th and early 20th centuries. It is only now being rediscovered. California psychiatrist and former National Institutes of Health researcher, Dr Tod Mikuriya, says, 'The power of cannabis to fight depression is perhaps its most important property' (Rosenthal, 1997; 58).

Marijuana can produce unpleasant feelings, such as paranoia, and other dysphorias (which means bad feeling, as opposed to euphoria which means good feeling). People who use marijuana regularly report that these bad feelings do diminish as they develop a familiarity with its effects. However, using marijuana to treat mood disorders can be very tricky. Since active mood disorders often warp one's observational skills, reports by patients about marijuana lifting them out of depression are inherently unreliable. If you intend to use marijuana for this purpose, it is very important that you thoroughly discuss it with your doctor. Patients who respond well report that marijuana not only diminishes their undesirable moods, it also motivates them to productivity. For some of these patients, depression was a by-product of a debilitating disease or illness for which marijuana provided a welcome remedy. For others, the marijuana seems to have acted directly on the depression.

The mental component of the pre-menstrual syndrome (PMS) often causes psychological problems and is now technically classified as an atypical (not typical) depression. Many women report benefit from using marijuana to improve the symptoms of PMS. In some societies, marijuana has long been used for this purpose. It seems to have the dual ability to reduce pain from menstrual cramps as well as deal with the atypical PMS depression.

Sexual Problems

There are widespread reports that marijuana is an aphrodisiac, that it promotes sexual arousal, enhances sexual pleasure, and helps individuals to overcome sexual inhibitions. On the other hand, many people report the opposite, that marijuana either has no effect on their sexuality or leaves them with a reduced interest in sex.

The claims that marijuana is a sexual stimulant come from both men and women, young and old. They are too numerous to dismiss. At the same time, as with so many other effects of marijuana, differences between individuals, and perhaps within the same individual at different times, may be more important than anything else in determining the impact of marijuana on sexuality.

Many patients using marijuana for problems other than their sexuality also report beneficial effects with respect to sex. Some of these patients have sexually related problems that are side-effects of other disorders. Many of them report that using marijuana to alleviate pain and suffering also results in improved sexual function. Other patients find that sexual performance is increased when their use of marijuana allows them to stop taking more debilitating drugs. For example, patients who normally take barbiturates often complain about reduced sexual responsiveness. When these patients substitute marijuana for the barbiturates, their sexual problems often disappear.

It is not likely that we will benefit from any scientific studies on this subject any time soon. For one thing, if marijuana's effect on sexuality is primarily a psychological rather than physiological phenomenon, it will be very difficult to conduct controlled scientific studies. Scientists cannot look inside the minds of their subjects and control or account for all possible influences on a sexual response at a particular time. For that reason, it will never be possible to definitively conclude that marijuana is a sexual stimulant.

In the meantime, with increasing demand for Viagra and other chemically based sexual stimulants, it is clear that large numbers of people are ready to try some kind of drug therapy for what they believe to be their sexual problems. Before taking drugs that might have harmful side-effects, such people might want to try marijuana. The only way to be certain whether it will work or not is to experiment, as it is clearly not effective for everyone.

No doubt, there are other conditions, not included in this chapter, for which patients are using marijuana. As the health benefits of marijuana become better known, more and more patients will seek those benefits and new information about marijuana will become available to the rest of us. Hopefully, renewed interest in the medicinal properties of marijuana will also encourage the federal government to relax the severe limitations it has placed on scientists trying to do clinical research on the drug. Marijuana has great potential for patients. All that stops it from making a far greater contribution to medicine than it already has is its continuing status as an illegal plant.

Chapter 16
Health Dangers of Marijuana: Some Real, Some Not

Marijuana is a drug, and any drug brings with it an element of risk. However, the actual risk is far less severe than some of the lurid rumours about the dangers of its use. More is being discovered every year about how marijuana works in the body and just what risks patients take in using it. Whether you are new to the medical use of marijuana, or someone who has tried it before, either for medical or recreational purposes, you will want to separate the risks from the rumours. In this chapter, we will try to address some of the questions about health risks of marijuana that people most commonly ask about.

If you are interested in a more thorough discussion of the health risks that may or may not be associated with marijuana use, the three best books on the subject are *Marijuana Myths, Marijuana Facts* by Lynn Zimmer, PhD, and John Morgan, MD, *Marijuana, The Forbidden Medicine* by Lester Grinspoon, MD, and *Cannabis in Medical Practice* edited by Mary Lynn Mathre, RN. All can be ordered at bookshops in the UK, or from www.Amazon.com on the Internet.

Marijuana and Cardiovascular Performance

In most people, marijuana tends to lower blood pressure and increase heart rate, usually very slightly. Both effects typically last for about 30 to 90 minutes, the same period that the high is most noticeable. Neither effect is considered substantial enough nor reliable enough to be medically significant. Nevertheless, people with risk factors in these areas should be careful when using marijuana. Such patients would be wise to consult a doctor before smoking marijuana regularly.

Marijuana Smoke and Lung Damage

Smoking is certainly an unusual way to take medicine into the body. Critics of medical marijuana often cite this novel aspect of its use to ridicule the very idea that marijuana can have medicinal effects at all. However, the best way to take some drugs is by inhalation of a vaporized or aerosolized preparation, such as in the treatment of asthma. For many people, especially those suffering from nausea, smoking is the best way to use marijuana. Since we all know that tobacco smoke is harmful, isn't marijuana smoke harmful, as well?

The short answer is, yes, the smoke from marijuana, like any other smoke, can introduce harmful compounds into the lungs. These include smoke by-products like tars, as well as some of the approximately 460 components of marijuana which, when burned, may also produce harmful substances. There is the possibility that some of these compounds can build up, not only in the lungs, but also in the mouth, the throat and the air passages leading to the lungs. It would be logical to assume that the more smoke taken into the lungs, the more likely it is that some damage will occur. However, the likelihood of actual damage must be assessed against the amount of smoke consumed and the body's ability to deal with or repair any damage.

Lungs are quite efficient at cleaning themselves. This is necessary given the normal amount of soot, dust, smog and other impurities we breathe into our lungs in the course of our daily lives. However, this capacity can be overwhelmed, as is amply demonstrated in the case of tobacco smokers. Recent evidence suggests that even the very modest amounts of tobacco smoke inhaled second-hand can cause damage to nonsmokers.

In most cases, typical marijuana smokers will consume far less smoke than typical tobacco smokers will. However, this is not an automatic safeguard against smoke damage from marijuana. Most medicinal marijuana use is limited to several puffs per day, or several puffs a few times per day. In either case, this amount of smoke is far less than what is consumed by tobacco users and probably means that the dangers are proportionately less. Medical marijuana users, who smoke several marijuana cigarettes daily, are in a different category. These patients must assess the risk from smoke damage versus the health benefits derived from using marijuana.

When discussing dangers of inhaling tobacco or marijuana smoke, lung cancer is the most serious complication. Marijuana smoke contains some chemicals known to cause cancer, including benzopyrene. Because of the lack of research on marijuana, no long-term studies have been done comparable to those that have looked at lung cancer and tobacco smoke. As a result, it is best to take a cautious approach and assume that too much marijuana smoke, like too much tobacco smoke, may create some risk of lung cancer.

One research study at UCLA has been monitoring heavy marijuana users for the past 15 years. These are people who have smoked an average of three to four marijuana cigarettes a day over that period. Since this is not a controlled experiment, firm conclusions are not possible. However, while none of these heavy marijuana smokers had lung cancer, their lungs did show some precancerous changes indicating some risk from heavy use (Zimmer and Morgan, 1997; 115).

The same UCLA study looked at other respiratory damage. In their conclusion, the researchers state, 'in contrast to the accelerated decline in lung function that occurs in tobacco smokers . . . findings in the present study do not support an association between even heavy, regular marijuana smoking and the development of chronic obstructive lung disease.' Chronic Obstructive Lung (or Pulmonary) Disease (COLD or COPD) describes airflow abnormalities in people with asthma, bronchitis or emphysema. The same study also concluded, based on examination of the airways of marijuana smokers, that 'marijuana smokers probably will not develop emphysema' (Zimmer and Morgan, 1997; 114).

In the UK, GW Pharmaceuticals, the company that has been given the licence to grow marijuana for research purposes, has developed a special inhaler device for taking measured amounts of cannabis. The BMA supports the cannabis research, but believes that cannabis smoking is harmful to health. It wants to see the development of 'targeted' medicines using cannabinoids.

There are two ways to possibly reduce smoke damage from marijuana. One is to use a filtering device, like a water pipe. However, while it is logical to assume that this would reduce the impurities in the inhaled smoke, there is no scientific evidence supporting that conclusion. We will describe how to use these devices in Chapter 20. The other way is to reject the advice commonly given to new marijuana users to hold the smoke in their lungs as long as possible. This advice assumes that the smoker's only objective is to have the body absorb as much marijuana as possible. At the same time, however, the tars and other impurities in the smoke are being deposited in delicate lung tissues. Two experts believe that most of the active ingredients in marijuana are absorbed almost immediately, and that the ill-advised practice of holding one's breath puts the smoker at greater risk of lung damage. They recommend inhaling and exhaling in a normal manner and not holding the marijuana smoke in the lungs for long periods (Zimmer and Morgan, 1997; 116).

Marijuana and the Immune System

Despite claims to the contrary by opponents of marijuana use, there is no evidence indicating that marijuana suppresses the human immune system. One study on guinea pigs showed increased rates of infection following doses of THC (Munson, 1983). However, to produce those increases the researchers had to administer doses up to one thousand times what is required to elicit a psychological reaction in humans. Other researchers, using skin tests that doctors employ to test immune responses in humans, found no difference between marijuana users and nonusers (Silverstein, 1976).

In 1981, at a conference jointly sponsored by Canada's Addiction Research Foundation and the World Health Organization, a scientific review of previous research on marijuana and immunity concluded, 'There is no conclusive evidence that cannabis (marijuana) predisposes man to immune dysfunction' (Munson, 1983). Later, when the US FDA approved THC (Marinol) as a prescription drug for use in cases of cancer chemotherapy, they found no evidence that it harmed the immune system. More recently, the FDA approved THC for use as an appetite stimulant for AIDS patients even though their immune systems are already compromised (Zimmer and Morgan, 1997; 109).

With respect to smoked marijuana, a study reported at the annual World AIDS Conference in 1996 compared two groups of HIV-positive men. One group was comprised of marijuana smokers while the other group was not. The marijuana smokers did not progress from being HIV-positive to having full-blown AIDS any faster than the nonsmokers, an indication that marijuana use had not put additional pressure on their immune systems (Di Franco, 1996).

A fungus called aspergillus can contaminate marijuana that has not been properly stored. This fungus presents a real risk to people with suppressed immune systems, like people with AIDS, because when inhaled it can cause aspergillosis, a serious lung infection. This disease does not occur in marijuana smokers whose immune systems are healthy, indicating that the fungus can be contained by the body's normal immune response. We will describe one method you can use to minimize the chance of using contaminated marijuana in Chapter 20.

The Effects of Marijuana on Reproduction and Sexuality

One group of researchers in 1974 found evidence of lower testosterone levels in men who were marijuana smokers. This finding gave rise to claims that marijuana had an adverse affect on sex hormones. However, many subsequent studies by other researchers were unable to duplicate these findings. They concluded that marijuana smoking, even at very high rates of consumption, had no impact on male sex hormones. The same 1974 study found lower sperm counts in male marijuana users. Once again, other studies failed to confirm this finding. At present, there is no convincing evidence that marijuana disrupts sexual or reproductive function or has any impact on human fertility rates (Zimmer and Morgan, 1997; 95).

There are numerous reports from a variety of cultures and countries around the world that marijuana can enhance sexual pleasure. However, if it does have aphrodisiac qualities, they differ widely from one person to the next. Some people report a reduced interest in sexual activity while high, while others claim the opposite. Given the complexity of the human sexual response and the degree to which it is affected by numerous psychological factors, the marijuana high is probably only enhancing whatever tendencies are already present. In any case, there are no scientific studies that bear on this issue one way or the other.

Marijuana and Addiction

Addiction is an important question on the minds of many patients first considering the medical use of marijuana. They want to know if they will be able to stop using marijuana once they start. The question is only important to patients who have never smoked marijuana before. Those with prior experience already know the answer.

Drugs made from the opium poppy are called opiate narcotics, or just opiates, and include heroin and morphine. These and other drugs, such as alcohol and tobacco, present a danger of physical and psychological dependence when used daily. When these drugs are abruptly stopped, an adverse reaction called withdrawal may occur. In regular opiate users, withdrawal can include crippling muscle spasms, profuse sweating, severe nausea and pain. In alcoholics, withdrawal symptoms can include shakiness, seizures, hallucinations (delirium tremens) and death. Long-term tobacco use is equally hard to break, but the withdrawal symptoms are far less severe. These symptoms can be relieved by taking more of the dependence-producing drug, getting medical treatment with different drugs, or by suffering through the withdrawal effects, a process called 'going cold turkey' that can last for days.

There is no indication that marijuana causes physical or psychological dependence. None of the ravages of physical or psychological dependence or withdrawal described above occur when marijuana users quit smoking or ingesting it. Marijuana users report being able to quit fairly easily, even if they have been smoking marijuana frequently for many years. Furthermore, most marijuana users find that they do not have to constantly increase the amount of marijuana they use in order to maintain the same effect. That is quite different from alcohol, opiates and tobacco, for which many regular users report the increasing need for larger amounts to achieve the desired result.

Nonetheless, some people who have consumed large amounts of marijuana over a very long time do report difficulty when they try to stop. The difficulty is limited to complaints like mild nervousness, irritability and trouble sleeping. Because these complaints are so dramatically different from those described above, researchers are not clear whether they represent physical or psychological dependence. Since marijuana can alter mood and consciousness when consumed in sufficient quantities, it may create a dependency that some people find hard to break. In any case, this kind of dependency affects only a small portion of marijuana users and is hardly comparable to the physical and psychological dependency that results from the use of addictive drugs like alcohol, opiates and tobacco (Mathre, 1997).

Marijuana and Memory

Marijuana disrupts short-term memory during the psychological high. The effect is mild, but clearly evident. While high on marijuana, the user has a tendency to forget some of what he or she may have said just moments before. This memory loss is not a complete blackout. Instead, it seems to randomly affect portions of prior dialogue or thinking. Most marijuana users are merely bemused at this phenomenon, but some, especially people new to the drug, find it unnerving. Marijuana seems to have no comparable impact on long-term memory. In addition to short-term memory loss, marijuana also disrupts concentration, especially on tasks that require some patience. Conversations tend to stray, people forget where they have put items, and if reading, they may find it difficult to recall material that they just read. The disruption of short-term memory and concentration disappears as the psychological high gradually ends, usually within 60 to 90 minutes. It leaves no long-term damage.

Given the disruption of memory and concentration, it is unwise to attempt any serious learning while under the influence of marijuana. This is why there is so much concern about schoolchildren and teenagers using marijuana. The focus required to do well in school would be difficult for anyone to maintain if their powers of short-term memory and concentration were regularly impaired.

Marijuana, Motivation and Performance

The loss of concentration while using marijuana makes it more difficult to perform detailed work or to follow through on commitments. For example, doing assembly line work that requires fine discrimination would suffer under the influence of marijuana. In addition, the tendency of marijuana to make some people sleepy would also reduce productivity. Since marijuana is mildly intoxicating, users should not drive while under its influence or undertake any tasks that require precise physical coordination, especially if they involve dangerous machinery.

Some concern has been raised about loss of motivation in frequent marijuana users. While this is a possibility, it is very difficult to come to firm conclusions one way or the other. Studies that report a correlation between marijuana use and loss of motivation (amotivational syndrome) in teenagers are unable to show that marijuana is the cause of the poor motivation (Zimmer and Morgan, 1997; 62–64). It is unclear if the apparent lack of motivation is caused by marijuana use, by underlying psychiatric disorders including depression or by social factors that, in turn, may contribute to marijuana use. The National Household Survey on Drug Abuse, published by the US Department of Health and Human Services in 1997, reports that social factors such as annual family income below $9,000 (about £6300) and lack of health insurance were associated with the highest prevalence of past-year marijuana use. In the UK, marijuana abuse is still more prevalent in lower income families.

Long-Term Marijuana Use

The books cited at the beginning of this chapter describe numerous long-term studies of heavy marijuana users. One study, done in New York in the 1940s, looked at users who had averaged seven marijuana cigarettes per day for eight years. There was no evidence of mental or physical decline in this population (LaGuardia Report, 1944).

More recently, three major studies were done in Jamaica, Greece and Costa Rica on very heavy marijuana users who had been smoking numerous marijuana cigarettes every day for years or even decades (Comitas, 1976; Carter, 1976; Boulougouris, 1976). They were drawn from subcultures in which marijuana is either part of a religious sacrament or is in frequent everyday use. Researchers compared the heavy marijuana users to nonusers. They found no evidence of intellectual or neurological damage, no personality changes, and no loss of motivation with respect to work or involvement with other people. Follow-up studies on the Costa Rican sample, done twelve and seventeen years after the original research there, continued to show no meaningful difference between the very heavy marijuana users and nonusers (Page, 1988).

Marijuana and Future Research

There are signs that the US government can be pressured into permitting more research on medical marijuana. Following the November 1996 passage of California's Proposition 215, which permits medical patients to use marijuana under state law, the federal government started to back away from its stubborn opposition to new marijuana research. The White House quickly announced that $1 million would be given to the National Academy of Sciences' Institute of Medicine to review existing knowledge on the effects of marijuana, both positive and negative. A month later, the National Institutes of Health (NIH) hosted a public scientific conference to discuss the existing scientific data and to recommend how new studies should be designed. Given that the NIH is a major source of funding for scientific investigations on a wide range of subjects related to health, a new wave of marijuana studies may now be a real possibility.

Nevertheless, there remains widespread scepticism about

the willingness of the US government to follow through on this possibility. Too many of its spokespersons, including the current federal drug Tsar, Barry McCaffrey, have belittled the medical uses of marijuana. Worldwide research is essential if marijuana use is to be accepted on a broad scale. While initiatives are under way in the UK, and there is widening support for the legalization of marijuana for medicinal purposes, it is unlikely that the UK government will make changes to the law unless there is more concrete research. Public scrutiny and ongoing press coverage of the medical marijuana issue may alter the equation and force some of these officials to make good on their promises. Likewise, more medical marijuana voter initiatives have the potential to keep public demand for access to medical marijuana strong enough to force new research.

Chapter 17
Why Is Marijuana Illegal?

By now you are probably wondering why and how marijuana became illegal in the first place. Volumes have been written about this question, each of which reflects, in varying degrees, the point of view of its author. We will try to give you our point of view, and hopefully you will try to remember that it is as biased as anyone else's. With respect to our society's laws, practices and beliefs about marijuana, there are many valid and legitimate points made by both proponents and opponents. There is also a good deal of nonsense.

Each side in the dispute cites data on public opinion and personal behaviour to support its views. On the one hand, we have laws that punish large-scale cultivation or sale of marijuana with many years in prison. These laws are supported by a clear majority of voters, and numerous attempts to repeal them have failed. On the other hand, poll after poll indicates that somewhere between one-quarter and one-third of our citizens believe that marijuana use, even for recreational purpose, should be legal. This is not a tiny minority that can be written off as a radical fringe. It is an enormous segment of our population, involving tens of millions of people. Furthermore, even the US government admits that there are probably about 70 million Americans who have tried this illegal substance at some point in their lives. A law broken by 70 million people may be in need of some revision. In the UK, that figure is nearly 6 million – a large proportion of the population. With 2.5

million regular users in the UK, there is a very clear message being sent to government officials.

The situation, some argue, is not unlike the period of Alcohol Prohibition (1920–33) in which Americans tried to ban the use of alcohol. It didn't work because too many people broke the law. That yardstick can be applied to drugs, as well. Today, much of the emotion behind the ban on illegal drugs is allegedly due to concern about teen drug use. But the most recent and reliable study of teen drug use, done by the University of Michigan's Institute for Social Research in 1997 and funded by the US government's National Institute on Drug Abuse, reveals that 42.4 per cent of 12th graders used some illegal drug other than alcohol and tobacco during the previous year. This statistic offers clear proof that punishing people for illegal drug use doesn't work any better than punishing them for illegal alcohol use did 70 years ago. Worse, the statistic makes evident that our strategy for preventing teen drug use has utterly failed to accomplish that goal.

In the UK, a five-year study with a group of 700 14-year-olds at eight schools in the North-west of England showed that around 3 of 10 18-year-olds are regular illegal drug users, and twice as many have tried illegal drugs. The authors of the study are critical of the government strategy on drugs: 'The important public policy issues – about how we deal with otherwise law-abiding young citizens caught with drugs in their possession, and how we ensure the health and safety of young people who use drugs – remains unresolved.'

Another 1995 survey found that close to half of all 16-year-olds had tried an illegal drug, and that drug experimentation is starting earlier, with 11- to 13-year-olds now trying drugs more often than before. Professor Howard Parker of the University of Manchester claims that 'Cannabis dominates young people's drug use and it is with this drug's use that we need to grapple. I personally would want to see a drugs cautioning system for personal use, which is basically decriminalized possession.' He claims that the 'war on drugs' approach failed to distinguish between drugs. By failing to distinguish between cannabis and heroin, society was failing to protect early adolescents from a 'return of heroin'.

In this chapter, we'll try briefly to explain how this strange situation came about.

Criminalizing Marijuana in the US (1900–1937)

In the early 1900s, many Americans objected to the unregulated use of over-the-counter medicines. Marijuana was one such drug and its unregulated use was also criticized. In addition, there were reports that African Americans and Hispanic Americans and immigrants were using marijuana for recreational purposes, and that such use was leading to various behaviours defined as antisocial by the dominant white society. These perceptions have to be judged in the context of the rampant racism directed towards both groups at that time.

El Paso, Texas, passed the first ordinance prohibiting the sale and possession of marijuana in 1914. It soon became a national trend. By the early 1920s, marijuana was banned in states across the country, but federal legislation on marijuana lagged behind. Various campaigns were then launched to create a federal ban on marijuana. In 1937, just a few years after the repeal of Alcohol Prohibition, these efforts succeeded in passing the Marihuana Tax Act (the drug is sometimes spelled with an 'h') which made it a crime to use marijuana.

Harry Anslinger, a Prohibition law enforcement officer, had become director of the Department of the Treasury's Bureau of Narcotics shortly after Prohibition ended. Anslinger and his staff saw marijuana as the next great threat to America, and beginning in the early 1930s, the Bureau lobbied hard to associate marijuana with crime. Anslinger formed an alliance with William Randolph Hearst, the newspaper tycoon, who frequently published lurid stories about heinous crimes allegedly committed under the influence of marijuana. Historical research has revealed that the entire effort had more to do with selling newspapers and building political opposition to marijuana than reporting the truth.

For example, in one case, Anslinger falsely claimed that a 21-year-old boy, Victor Licata, of Tampa, Florida, had killed his family under the influence of marijuana. Licata had been diagnosed with a severe mental disorder the year before the 1933 murders and had tried marijuana six months later, but no evidence ever showed that he had used marijuana at the time of the killings. At one point, Anslinger called marijuana 'the most violence-producing drug in the history of mankind', and said its use was 'reducing thousands of boys to criminal insanity'. Hearst and other tabloid sensationalists were only too happy to distribute these falsehoods. They led in turn to other false but sensational propaganda, like the film, *Reefer Madness*, which purported to demonstrate that normal citizens could be corrupted by marijuana. Thus, the stage was set for passage of the 1937 Marihuana Tax Act.

Marijuana Re-enters the US Culture (1950s to 1970s)

The use of marijuana as a medicine virtually disappeared during the 1940s and early 1950s. Recreational use was driven underground in this period, as well, but such use continued within subcultures already familiar with it. By the mid-1950s, jazz musicians and 'Beat Generation' poets and writers, among others, began openly to discuss their affinity for the drug. This affected college-aged youth, especially on some of the nation's more progressive campuses, and by the early 1960s, many students had begun to experiment with marijuana.

It was then that a series of cultural explosions shook American society and opened what became a huge rift between young adults and their elders. The advent of the birth control pill dramatically changed sexual behaviour. Rock and roll and folk music created a subculture that isolated many young Westerners from older citizens. The war in Vietnam led millions of American students to question their loyalty to a society and a nation waging what they saw as an unjust and brutal war of aggression. All of this combined to alienate many young people from societal norms, one of which was to avoid the use of marijuana. Smoking the drug became a sign of youthful rebellion, and the 1960s triad of sex, drugs and rock and roll captured a generation.

Marijuana came out of the closet. Students and young people smoked it openly and defiantly. They criticized the hypocrisy of the older generation for consuming a more harmful and addictive drug, alcohol, while making it a criminal offence to use marijuana. A rebellious subculture emerged which was symbolized by marijuana use. It stood for peace not war, instant gratification instead of sacrifice and careful planning for the future, sex over abstinence, and rebellion against authority of all kinds. Marijuana use was a rite of initiation and an ongoing sacrament for this subculture. Its point of view directly contradicted the mainstream puritanical values of the larger society, and a cultural chasm tore through the Western world.

That gap has yet to fully close, as the generation of the 1960s and early 1970s continues to hold more liberal and tolerant views on many issues than the rest of the nation. Although it is somewhat of an overgeneralization to say so, the two sides in the modern dispute over marijuana have their roots in this cultural divide. Many who advocate more liberal policies on marijuana today were part of the youth culture of yesterday. And many who now support severe criminal penalties for marijuana use see the 1960s and the values that emerged from them as the beginning of a period of moral, religious and patriotic decay, the chief symptom of which was drug use.

With so many people in the 1960s and 1970s living in open defiance of the marijuana laws, some accommodation had to be made. Complete legalization lacked majority support. Instead, many US states reduced the criminal penalties for personal use of marijuana from felonies and misdemeanours, which carry potential jail time, to 'violations', which were no more serious than minor traffic offences. But they left in place felony punishments for large-scale sales, importation and cultivation of marijuana.

This so-called decriminalization allowed people to continue using marijuana provided they didn't become involved in commercial transactions and their use remained sufficiently discreet to avoid notice by the police. As the former participants in the youth culture aged, entered the work force and won a place in the larger society, marijuana soon followed. Tolerance of its use reached a high point during the late 1970s, and some thought that outright legalization would soon occur. Even President Carter, in a message to Congress in 1977, said,

> Penalties against possession of a drug should not be more damaging to an individual than the use of the drug itself; and where they are, they should be changed. Nowhere is this more clear than in the laws against possession of marihuana in private for personal use . . . Therefore, I support legislation amending Federal law to eliminate all Federal criminal

penalties for the possession of up to one ounce of marihuana. (Baum, 1996; 94–95).

It was during this period that American health agencies began to permit a few patients to obtain marijuana for medical use from government supplies being grown for research purposes.

But a backlash was brewing. More and more children began using marijuana as a result of its increasing acceptance by personalities in the media and entertainment. Outraged parents joined other marijuana opponents and organized themselves to halt the 'normalization' of marijuana in mainstream society. The antimarijuana movement became a self-proclaimed 'parents' movement', which effectively argued that public policy should not be based on tolerance of marijuana use by adults, but rather on limiting its access to children.

'Un-selling' Marijuana in the US (1980s and 1990s)

The election of President Reagan in 1980 ended the slow trend towards liberalizing marijuana policy. In 1982, Reagan announced that his administration was 'taking down the white flag of surrender' toward illegal drugs, especially marijuana. By 1986, First Lady Nancy Reagan had coined her slogan 'Just Say No', as an antidrug message for kids and made antidrug work her personal priority. That same year, a group of media executives and business leaders formed the Partnership for a Drug-Free America, whose stated goal was to 'un-sell' drugs through the production and placement of public service ads in newspapers, on radio and on television.

Much of the new concern about illegal drugs was triggered by fears of cocaine use, which dramatically increased when 'crack' cocaine, a version that could be smoked in pipes, became widely distributed. Crack was frequently associated with gang violence. The wealth that many gangs accumulated selling crack spread the violence and led to police corruption and a dramatic escalation of heavy weaponry into urban areas across the country.

Despite the overwhelming problems with crack, most of the television ads sponsored by the Partnership for a Drug-Free America focused on marijuana. This was done because of the belief that marijuana was a 'gateway' drug that often led to cocaine and crack use. One ad featured a device monitoring the brain activity of a 'normal 14-year-old', with several pens moving energetically over a roll of paper. Then viewers saw the same device with only flat lines being drawn by the pens. The announcer claimed the device was now monitoring the brain of a 14-year-old who had smoked marijuana. Of course, the ad was not true. Journalists enquiring about it discovered that the device in the second part of the ad was not hooked up to anything at all and the ad was eventually withdrawn.

Similar distortions were incorporated into other ads. At the same time, programmes educating schoolchildren about the dangers of drugs achieved widespread distribution. Like the ads, these programmes focused disproportionately on marijuana, since it was the drug most commonly used by kids. Looking back on these advertisements and school programmes today, many observers believe they did little good. The problem, they argue, is that kids were not told the truth about marijuana. Given its widespread use among secondary school students, it was easy enough for users and nonusers alike to learn that marijuana was relatively benign compared to the harder drugs and alcohol. When the ads and school programmes exaggerated the dangers of marijuana, many kids simply wrote off the other, more critical, information they were getting about the dangers of cocaine, heroin and LSD. Some social analysts argue that these untruthful antimarijuana messages may have actually increased hard drug use among teens because they undercut the credibility of all antidrug messages (Rosenbaum, 1996).

The American message swept around the world, and 40 years of US propaganda had the desired effect: cannabis was considered to be a dangerous drug, and laws around the world were stiffened to prevent its sale, production and use.

Cannabis History in the UK

The medicinal use of marijuana in Britain and her colonies had a long and varied history. As long ago as the seventeenth century, the noted medieval herbalist, Nicholas Culpeper (1616–1654), listed a variety of medical uses of the common European hemp (*Cannabis sativa*), including anti-inflammatory, analgesic and antiparasitic activity. Culpeper made no mention of the psychotropic activity, although the temperate hemp he described would normally be of low drug content and be grown for fibre. Marijuana was considered to be a useful plant, like so many herbs, and was successfully used in folk medicine throughout Britain and, in particular, her Empire.

There was not much openly recreational drug use in Victorian England, other than alcohol. This was an age which demanded refinement, in every sense of the term. They took extracts, tinctures, distillations or the 'active ingredients' of traditional medicinal plants, sometimes in high doses. Cannabis was not considered to be a drug, although its merits were widely cited by both laymen and medical experts across

British history. The distinction between drug use and abuse had not been invented, and many patent medicines included cannabis (as well as opium and alcohol). In the 1840s, attempts were made to grow hemp for medicine in the London suburb of Mitcham. Experimenters used it for asthma and other chest problems, sleeplessness especially in cases of opiate or alcohol withdrawal, and with opium and bromide of potassium in treating insanity.

In the late 1830s, Dr William B. O'Shaughnessy, a physician at the Medical College of Calcutta, learned of cannabis and began experimenting with various cannabis preparations. He determined the drug was safe and effective in treating rabies, rheumatism, epilepsy and tetanus. O'Shaughnessy published his studies in a 40-page article entitled 'On the preparations of the Indian Hemp or Gunjah' in 1839. This marked the beginning of an intensive period of study throughout Europe and America. More than 100 articles were published between 1840 and 1900.

Attempts were made to isolate the active ingredient, but there were problems getting supplies of reliable strength, and confusion about different products from the same plant. It was, however, used to treat many disorders. In 1889, Dr E. A. Birch described in the *Lancet* the successful use of *cannabis indica* in the treatment of chloral hydrate and opium withdrawal, drawing attention to the abolition of craving and the anti-emetic (vomit suppressing) effects and the stimulation of appetite in patients who would not normally eat, or keep down, their food. Queen Victoria's personal physician, J. R. Reynolds, described it in 1890 as 'one of the most valuable medicines we possess'. In another *Lancet* article published in 1890, he described the use of *cannabis indica* for treating insomnia in the senile, acholic delirium, neuralgia, migraine, spastic paralysis and convulsions. Cannabis tincture and an extract made from resin were available wholesale through the Society of Apothecaries by 1871. Chemists extracted cannabene, cannabin tannin, cannabinnene and a variety of other confusing 'ingredients', but they had no idea which, if any, was the 'active ingredient' until cannabinol was isolated in 1895.

In the early 1900s a British Medical Association campaign against 'Secret Remedies' got most of the opiates, cocaine and cannabis out of tonics and non-prescription medicines. Doctors became responsible for most drug distribution as the consumer beverage trade withdrew. As drug dispensing was professionalized, substances used for self-medication were replaced by more refined, more medically controllable drugs.

In the UK, marijuana was quite openly used, particularly by the creative sectors of society, and it was not considered to be a threat to moral propriety or health until the scare stories began to filter in from the US. The Americans saw drugs of any type, including alcohol, as a modern scourge, and they claimed that they were debasing society at every level. They advocated complete prohibition of all intoxicants, including marijuana, and for 40 years encouraged the rest of the world to join them.

After a few scare stories of their own, involving cocaine and other opiates, the British began to accept the American intolerance. The *Daily Express* ran a series of articles lambasting the habits of degenerate circles, and included eating 'hashish' as one of their many sins. Before, during and after Prohibition, the US lobbied for international drugs laws, mixing economic self-interest with moralism. The Hague Conference in 1912 agreed to the principle of certain drugs being strictly for 'legitimate medical purposes'. It was never effective internationally because of obstruction by the British opiate and German cocaine businesses. The conference suggested an investigation of hemp, but it wasn't followed up.

Cannabis became illegal in the UK after the country agreed

the 1925 Geneva International Convention on Narcotics Control. There was hardly any parliamentary debate before it came into law as amendments to the Dangerous Drugs Act on 28 September 1928. Despite this, cannabis convictions were minor, and the drug was still used medicinally as required.

After the Marihuana Tax Act of 1937 in the US, American politicians initiated several international treaties and conventions that were aimed at controlling the drug trade. Signatories to these conventions agreed to pass laws prohibiting the possession, distribution and supply of a wide range of substances. Countries that had used cannabis as medicine or traditional social ritual for thousands of years found that they had to make a choice between political or economic stability, or marijuana.

In 1950 for the first time there were more prosecutions for cannabis than for opium and manufactured drugs together. That year a series of police raids on jazz clubs produced stories about 'black men with drugs' and 'white women', which drew cannabis into the league of 'dangerous' drugs.

Marijuana use experienced a renaissance in the 1960s, and it became the trademark of the 'hippy' generation. The question of legalization was first raised in this decade, and *The Times* published a full-page advertisement that argued that 'the law against marijuana is immoral in principle and unworkable in practice'. It was signed by many cultural icons of the day, including David Dimbleby, Bernard Levin and the Beatles. The advertisement caused such a stir that the government appointed a Home Office Select Committee to examine the arguments.

The Select Committee, which was chaired by Baroness Wootton, examined all of the available scientific evidence and made a number of suggestions. It concluded that 'There is no evidence that this activity is causing violent crime or aggression, anti-social behaviour, or is producing in otherwise normal people conditions of dependence or psychosis requiring medical treatment. The report suggested that while it was probably necessary to continue to restrict the availability of cannabis, it was a mistake to regard cannabis as similar to heroin and cocaine. The committee recommended that possession should no longer be regarded as a serious crime and imprisonment should no longer be viewed as an appropriate penalty in cases of possession.

By the time the Wootton report came out, the Conservatives had been replaced by a new Labour government which rejected the Wootton recommendations. In 1971, Sunny Jim Callaghan, then Home Secretary, introduced the Misuse of Drugs Act, which remains in force today. Until the late 1960s, doctors were able to legally prescribe Tincture of Cannabis, a product that is no longer on the market. Although opiates and other narcotics were still used in medicine, cannabis was banned, largely because inadequate research into its effects had taken place.

New research proposals are, however, promising. The British Medical Association recently published a major report on the therapeutic uses of cannabis. *Therapeutic Uses of Cannabis* draws a distinction between recreational misuse and using the drug to relieve pain. The report acknowledges that thousands of people resort to taking cannabis illegally in an attempt to ease their distressing symptoms, for example, glaucoma, muscle spasms, chronic pain and nausea.

The report includes moving accounts from individual patients who have used cannabis in desperation when conventional drugs have failed them. However because of the current state of the law, much of the evidence from those claiming relief is anecdotal.

The BMA report *Therapeutic Uses of Cannabis* examines the

scientific evidence for the wider medicinal use of cannabinoids – derivatives of cannabis – for a range of medical problems: nausea and vomiting associated with cancer chemotherapy, muscle spasticity, pain, anorexia, epilepsy, glaucoma, bronchial asthma, mood disorders and psychiatric conditions, and hypertension.

The report underpins the policy of the BMA that certain additional cannabinoids should be legalized for wider medicinal use. It sets the research agenda and identifies the legal steps that need to be taken before new treatments can be developed.

The report recommends further research including investigating the long-term effects of cannabinoids on chronic conditions. To facilitate research, the BMA recommends a change in the law. It suggests that advice should be given from the World Health Organisation (WHO) to the United Nations Commission on Narcotic Drugs to reschedule certain cannabinoids under the United Nations Convention on Psychotropic Substances. The Home Office could then amend the Misuse of Drugs Act in response. If WHO feels unable to give such advice, the Government should consider changing the Misuse of Drugs Act to allow cannabinoids to be prescribed to patients with particular medical conditions whose symptoms are being inadequately controlled under present arrangements. A central registry should be kept of those patients to allow follow-up of long-term effects.

The government responded by allowing research into the medicinal effects of marijuana to commence, and studies are currently under way.

Fears about Marijuana Use Today

Many Westerners, including those who came of age in the 1960s, have retreated from their earlier acceptance of marijuana. They are asking questions about its long-term effects on health and motivation, and its impact on children and teenagers. Alongside these general concerns is the belief that recent advances in marijuana cultivation have led to a more potent and dangerous substance than was in general distribution just a decade ago. In addition to these questions and concerns, our society has yet to resolve the cultural cleavage that took place in the 1960s. Marijuana remains a symbol of this cleavage, as opponents of its use continue to associate it with hedonism and irresponsibility, while advocates claim that its continued illegality exemplifies an oppressive and intolerant society.

We covered specific concerns about marijuana and health in Chapter 16. We will now briefly address some of the other fears about marijuana below.

Marijuana is much more potent, and therefore more dangerous, today than it was a decade ago. We often hear that today's marijuana is 20 to 30 times stronger than what was smoked in the 1960s and 1970s. This message is often directed at parents who may have experimented with marijuana in college, but are being warned about allowing their children to smoke it today. While high potency marijuana was certainly available in the 1960s, it is probably true that more of it is in distribution today. However, strangely enough, this results in certain advantages as well as dangers.

There is no doubt that if one smokes the same amount of high potency marijuana as low potency marijuana, a more intense psychoactive reaction will take place. Potency is generally defined in terms of the concentration of THC. Since THC is a psychoactive substance, the more of it taken into the body, the more powerful the high that results. If a large amount of high potency marijuana is smoked by an unsuspecting person, like a teenager, who must then perform a difficult task, like driving a car or taking an exam, serious consequences can result.

On the other hand, the higher potency of the marijuana can also mean that its desired effects can be attained by smoking less. One aspect of smoking marijuana that is clearly unhealthy is the simple act of inhaling smoke. While it does not contain nicotine as tobacco does, marijuana does contain tars that can damage lung tissue. Higher potency marijuana allows people to cut down their intake of smoke while getting the same amount of THC. Patients, especially those concerned about their respiratory health, may find it beneficial to pay for higher potency marijuana, which is more expensive, because they can use less of it to achieve the desired effects. In any case, patients should always be aware of the potency of the marijuana they are using.

Marijuana is a 'gateway' to the use of harder drugs. Some argue that marijuana users will soon graduate to harder drugs like cocaine and heroin. This notion is advanced by the Center on Addiction and Substance Abuse (CASA), an American antidrug organization, following a survey of drug users they conducted. Based on their survey results (Califano, 1994), this group concluded that marijuana users were 85 times more likely to go on to harder drugs than those who did not use marijuana. The survey actually showed that only 17 per cent of marijuana users went on to try harder drugs, while 83 per cent did not. Only 0.2 per cent of cocaine users had never tried marijuana. CASA divided 17 per cent by 0.2 per cent and the result is 85. The 85 number is large not because the majority of marijuana users go on to hard drugs. The number is large because it is rare for people to try cocaine without trying marijuana first (Zimmer and Morgan, 1997; 35–37). The study actually shows that people who use uncommon drugs such as cocaine and heroin, try common drugs (tobacco, alcohol and marijuana) first. Virtually all of the marijuana users had also used alcohol and tobacco.

In the UK, there are roughly 6 million cannabis users, and nearly 300,000 hard drug users. Five years ago, there were roughly 5 million cannabis users . . . and nearly 300,000 hard drug users. While cannabis use is clearly on the increase, hard drug use is not.

It is hard to argue that marijuana use leads to hard drug use when 83 per cent of marijuana users do not go on to other drugs. On the other hand, the study does present evidence that while marijuana use may not cause hard drug use, it is associated with a greater likelihood of hard drug use. The question is, why? There are two likely answers. First, the same dealers often sell marijuana and hard drugs. Thus, in obtaining marijuana, some users are exposed to opportunities to purchase hard drugs that nonusers do not encounter. Second, both marijuana and the hard drugs share an outlaw mystique. As a result, people looking for ways to rebel against authority are drawn to both, much as others are attracted to forbidden fruit.

Marijuana may damage children while they are still growing and may reduce their overall motivation. This claim is very difficult to address as no scientific data has been collected that would allow us to give a definitive answer. Furthermore, it is unlikely that such data ever will be collected. To do so would mean comparing two groups of children, one given marijuana, the other not, over a period of many years. No responsible scientist would permit such a comparison. The next best thing would be to perform animal studies to address some of the health and developmental implications. However, such studies would fail to answer questions about motivation or other psychological phenomena.

Thus the safest course, and one that virtually everyone on both sides of the marijuana issue will readily support, is to prohibit recreational marijuana use by children. As a society, we have clearly failed to do that, just as we have failed to prohibit illicit alcohol and tobacco use by children. In fact, surveys reveal it is often easier for a child to obtain marijuana than alcohol (although both are illegal for children). Some think that dealers prefer to sell to children because youngsters are unlikely to be undercover cops looking to 'sting' the dealer. As long as we continue to keep marijuana illegal and the underground market profitable, we may indirectly be encouraging sales to children. Thus far, our society has relied primarily on the tactics of instilling fear and threatening punishment to limit access to marijuana. Perhaps it's time to place far greater emphasis on accurate and meaningful education to protect our children.

The Role of Marijuana in the Larger 'War on Drugs'

Patients have every right to ask why governments cling so stubbornly to the notion that medical marijuana should be illegal. The answer is not hard to find. Officials have stated over and over again that they see the legalization of marijuana for medical use as a first step towards its legalization for recreational use. We would like to think that they have no idea how many hundreds of thousands of patients they are condemning to a life of unnecessary pain and suffering by taking that position. Unfortunately, the evidence points in the opposite direction.

How then can we explain this callous disregard for these patients? It must have more to do with marijuana itself than with a system of controls over dangerous medicines. After all, doctors are permitted to prescribe morphine, cocaine and amphetamines, all drugs that are highly addictive and potentially lethal. Why not marijuana, which is neither?

The answer may lie in the size and scope of the 'War on Drugs'. In the US, they currently invest a massive amount of money in this effort, roughly $16 billion per year out of the federal budget and a similar amount from state and local budgets. In the UK, an estimated £380 million was spent on proactive antidrugs activity in 1997/8. That figure will jump by another £188 million by the year 2000. However, those totals are just the direct governmental expenditures. They do not include all the drug-testing programmes, the drug education programmes and the drug rehabilitation programmes. A sizable portion of our national economy is spent either directly or indirectly waging the war on drugs. A huge number of people, from police officers and prison guards to laboratory technicians and drug educators, are employed in this effort. Enormous amounts of capital have been invested in prison construction, testing laboratories, school programmes, surveillance technology and so forth. Profits are made from all of these investments. The war on drugs has become a very big business.

Many people are surprised to learn that about 80 per cent of this big business is focused on the soft drug, marijuana, while only about 20 per cent deals with the hard drugs, like heroin and cocaine. In the 1950s, before widespread use of marijuana, there were about 500,000 heroin addicts in the United States. Budget allocations for dealing with this problem were only a tiny fraction of what we spend now. Today, there are still about 500,000 heroin addicts in the United States. These figures are echoed in the UK, where there are about 160,000 heroin addicts, much the same number as there have always been, despite the huge sums spent fighting drug abuse. However, the war on drugs has mushroomed into a multi-billion dollar colossus primarily because of the extent to which they have criminalized marijuana use. As an example, in 1996 alone, the FBI reports that there were over 600,000 Americans arrested for marijuana use. In the UK, in 1995, of 93,631 drug offences, almost 77,000 of those were for cannabis.

With dozens of billions spent per year to feed the war on drugs, it is no wonder that governments have a strong bias in favour of continuing current policy – despite the fact that this policy is such a massive and self-evident failure. If marijuana were to be legalized for recreational use, some 80 per cent of those billions would be lost to the individuals, businesses and government and nongovernment programmes receiving that money. This may explain why there is so much political force deployed today to keep marijuana illegal, and why patients who want to use it strictly for medical purposes have become mere pawns in the game.

It may first appear that this is merely a liberal point of view. However, many well-known conservatives hold similar views. Television personality, William F. Buckley, publisher of *The National Review*, a leading conservative publication, devoted the better part of his 12 February 1996 issue to a feature entitled 'The War on Drugs is Lost'. It contained essays by Mr Buckley and six others. One was written by Joseph McNamara, a former New York City policeman who later was chief of police in Kansas City, Missouri, and San Jose, California. Mr McNamara's essay begins, 'It's the money, stupid' (McNamara, 1996).

Leaders on the left and right agree. This titanic war on drugs is no longer a means to solve a problem but now has become an end in itself.

Chapter 18
What Is It Like To Be 'High'?

Polling data shows that almost half of the adults likely to be reading this book have smoked marijuana at least once in their lives. These people already know what it's like to be high. This chapter is written for everyone else.

Because marijuana is an illegal drug, there is a great deal of frightening information in circulation about its effects, both psychological and physical. Little of this information is actually true, as we will explain below. However, if you have never smoked marijuana before, you are likely to be a little nervous about first getting high. If you are careful, you need not be overly concerned. Marijuana is a mild intoxicant. The best way to begin using it is by smoking or eating a little at first in order to get used to its effects gradually, just as you might recommend to a person trying alcohol for the first time.

Marijuana is often placed in the same category as truly dangerous drugs like heroin and cocaine. In Chapter 16, we explained that this was quite inappropriate. The effect of marijuana on the mind and body is usually no more dramatic than that of a few glasses of wine. Of course, if you have never had a few glasses of wine, or any other alcoholic drink, you might be quite surprised at the intoxicating effect and be somewhat upset if you had not been warned to expect it.

The same is true of marijuana. You may have heard frightening stories about 'bad trips' and 'losing control' under the influence of marijuana. This happens on rare occasions when individuals are simply surprised by the high they are experiencing and have an anxiety attack at the thought that it might not go away. Fortunately, the marijuana high does dissipate rapidly. If one is predisposed to anxiety attacks, it is especially important to pay attention to the mind-set being brought to the experience and the setting in which the experience is taking place. If you relax, use the marijuana in a safe and familiar environment, perhaps with a trusted loved one at your side, and avoid situations in which fear and anxiety are likely to occur, the chance of your experiencing anything unpleasant is quite remote.

Before we describe what you should expect the first time you use marijuana, you should know that many patients report that marijuana used for medical purposes does not make them high at all. Patients fighting nausea, for instance, often need to take only a few puffs to deal with their nausea, and a few puffs may not be enough to produce any mental effects. Some patients simply do not get high, perhaps because they are not seeking that effect in the first place. You should also be aware that many people, whether they are recreational or medicinal users, report that they do not get high the first few times they try marijuana. It is only after several attempts that they begin to experience the high.

In any case, the mental and physical effects of marijuana wear off quickly, usually in 30 minutes to two hours if the marijuana is smoked and somewhat longer if it is eaten. Therefore, if your first experience with marijuana does turn out to be unpleasant, it is unlikely that the consequences will be any greater than having an unpleasant experience from drinking a little too much alcohol. There will be one difference, however. You will not have a hangover the next morning. Marijuana does not cause hangovers.

Mental Effects of Smoking Marijuana

The sensation of being high is quite subtle. Typically, it differs slightly from one person to the next and from one experience to the next. There is often a sense of amusement and well-being (euphoria). There is a feeling of relaxation and calm. People who are high often report that their awareness is heightened, their thinking a little more creative and loose. Sensations are heightened, too. Food seems to taste better. Music seems to sound better. The listener often reports being able to hear the complexity and nuances of the music more readily when high. Visual experiences may also be enhanced. People who are high seem to enjoy art, as well as the simple appearance of things, more profoundly than at other times. When marijuana produces effects like these, and the user is accustomed to the effects, it can be quite pleasurable, which helps explain why millions of people use marijuana solely for recreational purposes.

Thinking is slightly altered while high on marijuana. Individual ideas seem more interesting than they usually do and appear to be worth exploring from new and different angles. People occasionally become very fixated on specific thoughts, feelings or perceptions and want to talk about them in great, sometimes excruciating, detail. They feel a bit giddy about each new detail or idea they discover in this mental state, and will occasionally laugh out loud in reaction to the novel thoughts they are experiencing.

Nevertheless, with all of this seemingly heightened mental awareness comes some forgetting, as well. Marijuana impairs short-term memory. It has no effect on long-term, or permanent, memories. What this means in practice is that people who are high often cannot remember words they have just spoken or read. The sensation is similar to having something 'on the tip of your tongue' and not being able to remember it. Should that happen to you, do not be alarmed. Your short-term memory will be back to normal as soon as the high wears off. It seems that while high, the brain is unable to adequately record memories for recent events. At the same time, people who are high have no trouble remembering things that happened to them before becoming high.

In practice, the effect on short-term memory can lead to some amusing situations, as well as to some dangerous ones. For instance, while high, a person may decide to make spaghetti and put some water on the stove to boil. Before the water boils, the person is distracted by music playing in the next room, or by a desire to go outside and gaze at some flowers. Twenty minutes later, the person has forgotten about the spaghetti and the water boils merrily away.

If the activity subject to the short-term memory loss involves something more dangerous than making spaghetti, the results can be less amusing and far more serious. Activities having to do with fire, driving an automobile, caring for a child, or operating dangerous equipment can all have very serious consequences as a result of short-term memory loss. Lifeguards should not be high on the job; neither should people working on computer assembly lines. In general, activities that require close focused attention or physical coordination should not be undertaken while high.

Many people fear they will lose control of themselves if they get high on marijuana. For some, this is a fear of losing the normal inhibitions that keep them from acting out their impulses. People do becomes less inhibited when high, but the effect is usually far less pronounced than the loss of inhibitions while drunk on alcohol. Few people will engage in behaviours while high that they would not engage in otherwise. For example, unlike alcohol, and despite mistaken claims to the contrary, marijuana has no documented history of leading to violent behaviour.

Other people fear that marijuana might lead to some permanent impairment of their mental health. When they begin to experience mild anxiety while high, such fears intensify and can lead to increased levels of anxiety and a downward spiral into panic. The best way to avoid such a reaction is first to experiment with marijuana by gradually increasing the dose until you find the right amount and get more familiar with the experience of being high. In any case, keep in mind that the marijuana high is a very temporary experience, and one that the vast majority of users can easily adjust to, if not actually enjoy.

Some opponents of recreational marijuana use are so militant in their beliefs that they often stretch the facts beyond recognition. One example is their claim that marijuana can cause serious mental disorders, like schizophrenia. There is no evidence to support this claim. It is based on the story of one individual who was quite seriously disturbed before he tried marijuana, and found to be equally disturbed afterward. Another totally unfounded charge is that marijuana leads to violent behaviour, a claim based on political bias, not on the truth. In fact, marijuana is much more likely to calm a user's violent impulses.

Some naïve users worry that others will be able to tell when they are high. This can cause obvious concern when such worries are focused on police officers, employers or the users' own children from whom they may wish to keep their marijuana use hidden. This concern is only valid if you smoke an excessive amount. Once you get used to the experience, you will be able to control the amount of marijuana you take in and avoid unwanted and inadvertent disclosures of your marijuana use.

Physical Effects of Smoking Marijuana

Marijuana does cause some minor changes in physical function. People who smoke marijuana commonly feel that the mucous tissue in their mouth is excessively dry. Marijuana seems to take the moisture out of mucous membranes throughout the body, but this effect is most noticeable in the mouth. It is easily dealt with by drinking water.

People tend to eat more when high on marijuana. This effect has its therapeutic value for people who are too nauseous to eat or have a reduced appetite as a result of other clinical problems. However, the urge to eat when high will affect most people regardless of their medical condition. Most marijuana users report that food tastes considerably better when they are high, especially sweets. It is not clear whether this heightened sense of taste is what leads to increased appetite or whether the marijuana is having a more direct impact on appetite. In any case, expect to get a case of 'the munchies' when you are high. You might want to prepare for them by having some healthy snacks available and hiding the sweets, especially the chocolate, somewhere out of reach.

Marijuana can impede your coordination slightly. You should expect your reaction time to be a bit slow. Performing complex tasks requiring hand-eye coordination will be a little more difficult. However, unlike being drunk on alcohol, this effect will not cause slurring of speech, staggering or wild movements.

Some people have a heightened sensation of their hearts beating while high on marijuana. While it is true that marijuana does sometimes increase heart rate, the effect is small and quite temporary. Of course, if you have a history of heart problems, it would be wise to talk to your doctor before trying marijuana.

There are other, less common reactions to marijuana use. Some people get sleepy while high. In fact, the most common reaction to having smoked too much marijuana is to fall asleep. This effect is harnessed by some people who use marijuana to solve their sleep problems. Others may feel a heightened sense of touch, or may feel increased sensitivity in their skin. This is almost always pleasurable, and sometimes leads people who are high to enjoy a long hot bath or a massage. Not surprisingly, many people also experience increased sexual sensitivity while high.

As you can see, marijuana affects different people in different ways, both psychologically and physically. If you are careful and use common sense, you should have nothing to worry about. In all likelihood, the amount of marijuana you will need to alleviate your medical symptoms will not be great enough to induce a very pronounced high experience. Remember to avoid situations where you might be called upon to perform complex or potentially dangerous tasks. Begin experimenting with marijuana by using small amounts and then gradually increase them until you get the medical effect you want and, at the same time, become familiar with the high, which is actually a side-effect of the marijuana. If you do experience something unpleasant, keep in mind that it will last for only a brief period. On the other hand, if the side-effects you experience are pleasant and pleasurable, enjoy them. They're good for your health, too.

Chapter 19
How Do Patients Get Marijuana?

Regardless of its value as a medicine, the possession, sale and use of marijuana remains illegal under a variety of laws. That creates a very difficult situation both for patients who want to use it and for doctors who want to recommend it. Patients risk criminal prosecution if they are caught. Doctors risk various professional sanctions, such as the loss of their licence to practise medicine or the loss of their right to prescribe drugs. In the US, the Drug Enforcement Administration (DEA) has the authority to take away a doctor's prescription privileges if, in its view, the doctor abuses those privileges by helping patients obtain controlled substances like marijuana. Any doctor disciplined in this way would be unable to continue practising medicine. In the UK, no doctor can help to supply a patient with an illegal drug, and risks being struck off if he or she attempts to do so.

As a result, patients should not expect their doctors to help them get marijuana. Some doctors do not even feel free to recommend marijuana to their patients. In the US, DEA officials have threatened to pull the prescription privileges of doctors who merely recommend marijuana, but it is not clear they have a legal right to do so. A temporary federal court decision currently limits their ability to take such action in California (because of Proposition 215), but it is not clear whether this decision will be made permanent or will extend beyond California. Patients, of course, are free to question their doctors about marijuana, and doctors are free to respond to their questions. Nevertheless, the DEA does not want doctors to suggest marijuana use to their patients or to take any concrete steps to help them obtain it. No such action has been suggested in the UK, but there is no question that any doctor involved in obtaining drugs for patients would be subject to criminal prosecution.

Despite these constraints, many doctors are aware of the potential medical benefits of marijuana. They are willing to discuss it and do not object to patients using it. Other doctors have little or no knowledge about the medicinal uses of marijuana and may react with scepticism, or even anger, when patients mention the possible benefits of marijuana. You will have to decide how best to approach your own doctor. If he or she is unaware of the medicinal uses of marijuana, you might want to recommend one of the references listed at the end of this book. Try to understand the difficult position you may be putting your doctor in and act with patience and understanding. However, if your doctor refuses to work with you, then switch doctors. Your health is the most important issue.

We, as the authors of this book, face a similar problem. We cannot encourage you to violate the law. However, we have a free speech right to share information about the medicinal properties of marijuana with you, and we have done that in the earlier chapters of this book. In this chapter, we will exercise our free speech right to tell you how other patients and their loved ones have obtained marijuana in the past. You can draw your own conclusions. We are not recommending that you engage in any of these practices. Rather, we just want to make you aware of what others have done in situations that may be similar to yours.

In the stories told by other patients earlier in this book, you may have read about the social and personal conflict that can result from the stigma surrounding marijuana use in our society. This stress is of great concern to some patients and of little or no consequence to others. Fortunately, more and more patients, doctors, nurses and other healthcare providers are speaking out about their experiences with marijuana, in spite of its status as an illegal drug. This makes it easier for all patients who use it. It has also created a network of resources and support groups that you may be able to turn to for help. As you face important choices about your own medical treatment, in addition to talking to your doctor, you may want to seek contact with other patients who share your predicament. You may be able to find them through friendly nurses, marijuana buyers clubs, or on the Internet where you can communicate with patients around the world.

There are two ways patients obtain marijuana; they either buy it or grow it. If they buy it, they can do so in one of three ways. First, they can purchase it from someone known or recommended to them, like a friend or acquaintance, or the friend of a friend. Second, they can buy it at a marijuana buyers club (some are planned for the UK) or co-op created specifically to assist patients. Both these procedures entail relatively minimal risk. Third, marijuana can be purchased on the street from a stranger. This increases the risk dramatically. We will discuss each of these methods below.

Learn about the Marijuana Laws First

Since using or buying marijuana can place you or a loved one in legal jeopardy, you should first find out exactly what marijuana laws are in effect where you live. Because the laws on the books are not enforced in the same ways in different communities, you will also have to find out the actual police practices in your community. In some places, the law is enforced to the letter. In others, it is not. In many areas, individual police officers or district commanders simply look the other way when it comes to medical patients, regardless of overall policy or how strictly the laws are enforced with respect to the recreational use of marijuana.

It may not be easy to get the relevant information, but it will ease the stress you experience if you do. If you have a family solicitor, or a friend who is a lawyer, ask him or her to research the question for you. If you do not have access to a lawyer, you can check with local law enforcement officials yourself. Look in the phone book in the section on local government.

The laws affecting marijuana are clear, and over the past few years the UK government has been steadily increasing their control over this substance. The law concerning cannabis in the United Kingdom is the Misuse of Drugs Act 1971, which classifies cannabis as a class B controlled substance with no medicinal uses. This law defines a series of offences that you can be charged with relating to cannabis. The most common is possession.

You can be charged with possession of a class B drug if the police can prove the cannabis is or has been in your possession at any point, whether it was in your home, car or clothing. Possession implies that you were using the drug for personal use only, and is viewed less strictly than other drug-related offences.

More serious is the charge of possession with intent to supply, which takes place when the police believe you intended to sell or supply somebody else with cannabis. If they can prove that you did sell or supply marijuana you can be charged with supplying. Other marijuana-related charges that can be brought are unlawful production or trafficking. To enforce these laws the police have the power to stop, detain and search people on reasonable suspicion that they are in possession of cannabis.

Maximum sentences vary between the different charges. Possession is the least serious, and production is the most. The maximum sentence for possession of cannabis is 5 years in prison with a fine; occasionally people are let off with just a fine. Less serious offences are usually dealt with in magistrates courts where the maximum sentence does not exceed six months and/or a £5000 fine, or three months and/or fine for the least serious offences, which includes possession.

There is no question that parts of the UK are less strict about cannabis laws. A recent study showed that police forces across the country take very different approaches – unofficially, of course – towards cannabis. Many police forces in large cities will not bring individual cases of possession to court, and rely on a caution system instead. In other cases, some go even further and don't arrest people with small quantities of cannabis in their possession.

Smaller forces do, however, tend to take offences more seriously, and prison sentences are not uncommon. There is, however, call for reform of the cannabis laws by senior police officers.

The UKCIA (UK Cannabis Information) reported the details of a survey conducted among uniformed officers of various ranks. An anonymous questionnaire was sent out to a representative sample of 230 uniformed officers in the Sussex police force.

The survey was aimed at identifying the likelihood of arrest and prosecution following the apprehension of individuals in possession of small amounts of cannabis for personal use. The questionnaire also asked whether, either currently or before joining the police force, the officers had friends who used cannabis recreationally. Finally, various situational and personal variables were offered through which the officers could indicate the factors that would influence them towards or away from arresting an individual in possession of cannabis.

Of the total sample, 20 per cent already practise informal policing. This group were prepared to take no formal action when they felt the situation warranted none. A small minority of these officers responded by ignoring the offence altogether, but the majority handled it through an informal street caution.

The remaining 80 per cent of the sample reported acting formally against those found in possession of cannabis. In most cases this meant arrest and subsequent charges being brought against the individual.

Despite the more tolerant attitudes of some officers, cannabis offences continue to dominate the war on drugs. Indeed, 83 per cent of all drug offences in the UK during 1994 involved cannabis. The most common drug seizures involved less than 1 gram of cannabis. In the mid-1980s, less than 10 per cent of offenders were cautioned, about 50 per cent were fined, and 15 per cent were imprisoned. In an obvious relaxation of the laws, by the mid-1990s, more than 50 per cent were cautioned, about 20 per cent were fined and less than 10 per cent were imprisoned. However, over that period, the number of cannabis offences recorded jumped by more than 300 per cent (from 20,746 to 76,694). While the crime may be treated less seriously by officers and courts, there is no question that the laws are tightening.

Growing Your Own Marijuana

Patients who grow their own marijuana are able to generate a constant, low-cost supply of fresh marijuana. The marijuana they use will all come from the same strain and therefore will affect them in the same way with no surprises or disappointments resulting from variations in the strength or quality of the drug. On the other hand, such patients expose themselves to greater risk from law enforcement officials in the US, unless they live in California where cultivation by patients is legal under Proposition 215. As other states pass similar voter initiatives, this protection is likely to be extended.

New laws to ban the sale of cannabis seed and marijuana-growing equipment in the UK are being urged by police chiefs. The idea is being promoted by the Association of Chief Police Officers (ACPO), in an attempt to clamp down on the use and availability of cannabis.

At present home-growers are exploiting a legal loop-hole that allows them to buy cannabis seeds and the growing equipment legitimately from specialist shops and mail order. The cultivation of cannabis plants is illegal, but not the sale or purchase of seeds.

Colin Phillips, Chief Constable of Cumbria, and head of ACPO's drug committee, said he had raised the issue with Keith Hellawell, the new British 'drugs tsar', and would be urging Jack Straw, the Home Secretary, to introduce a new offence of possession of seed- and plant-growing equipment with the intention of cultivating cannabis.

There are an estimated 500,000 illegal cannabis plants being grown in Britain. Seeds cost from £40 to £70 for a packet of 10, depending on variety. Growing equipment, which includes trays and a lighting system, starts at £75.

Home-grown cannabis is becoming increasingly common, with 60 per cent of users having grown at least some of their own cannabis at some time. One in three growers used 'pedigree' types such as skunk or northern lights. Of those growing their own cannabis, 71 per cent were growing the plant indoors, 14 per cent in greenhouses and 23 per cent outdoors.

Techniques for growing marijuana have become very sophisticated in the past 20 years. It is beyond the scope of this book to bring together all of the information currently available on marijuana cultivation. We will try to suggest the basic questions patients need to ask, and outline the various ways cultivation can be approached.

However, any patient intending to grow marijuana for personal use should consult books, articles and magazines that focus on cultivation. Among the best are those written by Ed Rosenthal, Robert Connell Clarke or Mel Frank, listed in the back of this book. When you read the section in Chapter 20 on cooking with marijuana, you will see various websites where books on cultivation, as well as cooking, can be purchased. Cultivation books can also be found in many larger bookstores. *High Times*, a magazine for marijuana users, typically contains many articles and advertisements helpful to cultivators. It is available in most places with a large magazine selection.

One of the first questions a cultivator must answer is whether to grow the marijuana indoors or outdoors. Outdoor growing is simpler and cheaper. Marijuana grows like a weed. It thrives in all kinds of soils and environments and can be grown anywhere in the world depending upon the season. It is often no more complicated than planting the seeds and waiting for the marijuana to grow. Many patients sprout the seeds first by letting them sit in paper towels kept moist for several days. When white roots emerge from the seeds, they can be planted one inch into the soil with the seeds up and the roots down.

Unfortunately, there are risks associated with growing marijuana outdoors. Unless the plants are very well hidden in seldom-used areas, there is the risk of detection, either by thieves or by police officers. There is also the risk that animals, such as deer or foxes, will eat the plants. Protecting the plants from animals by using a fence increases the danger of detection.

Outdoor growing also means that the plants are susceptible to bacterial and fungal infection and insect infestation. In Chapter 20, we will explain how to sterilize marijuana to increase safety.

Growing marijuana indoors reduces the risk of detection and allows for cultivation any time of year regardless of the weather. It does require an investment in electrical equipment. At a minimum, this means indoor growing lights. At a maximum, it could also mean fans, meters, timers, soil, automatic watering devices and large amounts of electricity. This can entail purchases of anywhere from one hundred to several thousand dollars. The increased consumption of electricity can be dangerous as police narcotics squads often look for spikes in home electricity usage and search for hot spots in homes with infra-red detection equipment. Moreover, they tend to view well-run indoor growing facilities as the trade mark of a profiteer, even if the grower is just a capable medical patient. Finally, indoor plants are typically smaller, more frail and are still susceptible to infection and insects.

Whether marijuana is grown indoors or outdoors, it is usually best to separate the female plants from the male plants. The female plants produce the flowers, or buds, which contain the highest concentration of marijuana's active ingredients (cannabinoids). After drying, these buds can be smoked exclusively or in combination with dried leaves, but either way, they are preferable to the male plants because they have higher concentrations of active cannabinoids. Many cultivators kill all of the male plants early in the growing cycle. The remaining female plants are not fertilized, which means they do not produce seeds.

Seedless marijuana (*sinsemilla*) is preferred because it has a higher concentration of cannabinoids per weight of plant vegetation and it is time consuming to remove the seeds before smoking the buds. The seeds have been consumed as food for millennia but contain no active medicine, give off acrid smoke and may violently pop (like popcorn) when smoked. This popping, burning vegetation can land on one's body, clothes or furniture. Killing the male plants also reduces the number of plants under cultivation which may slightly reduce overall legal jeopardy.

The male plants can be allowed to survive if the cultivator wants the female plants to bear seeds for future planting or eating. If the male plants are killed, future planting can also be done from cuttings. As with many houseplants, a cutting (or 'clone') can be clipped off and rooted in water, then planted. An important advantage of using cuttings, or clones, is that the future plants will be identical to the plant from which the clipping came. In this way, a good strain can be found and cultivated over and over indefinitely.

Marijuana buds and leaves must be dried after they are harvested in order to properly prepare them for smoking. The various books and articles on marijuana cultivation will explain exactly when to harvest the plants and the various drying techniques. Many growers are only interested in the seedless buds from mature female plants, and that is usually all that is sold for medical or recreational purposes. However, patients growing for themselves often save the female leaves, as well. These can be smoked or baked into food. They still contain THC and other active ingredients in marijuana, but in much smaller concentrations than in the buds. Since exposure to smoke is undesirable, one can see that smoking a smaller amount of potent sinsemilla may allow one to get the desired medical benefits of marijuana with less smoke exposure. The same is true of any especially potent marijuana.

Patients new to marijuana cultivation often want to know how much they can get from a single plant. There is no easy answer to this question. Some new growers might harvest only an ounce of usable high-grade marijuana from a single plant. Those with more experience can get much more, especially from outdoor plants allowed to reach their full size, which can exceed eight feet in height. Law enforcement officials tend to view each plant as capable of producing a full pound (.4 kg) of marijuana, which is the main reason why growing any number of plants can get a cultivator into serious trouble.

Buying Marijuana

In most situations, the safest way for a medical patient to acquire marijuana is to buy it from a friend or acquaintance. Patients with little or no prior experience with marijuana tend to think that because they don't use marijuana, no one else they know does either. This is often not true. For example, most surveys estimate that about 13 million Americans will admit to having smoked marijuana in the past 30 days. In the UK, there are about 2.5 million or more. Cannabis is the UK's most popular illegal drug – by a long way. On average one out of every twelve adults with whom you are acquainted is likely to be a marijuana user.

This is an important number because it means that if you are a patient in need of marijuana, it might be easier for you to get it than you think. If you can become comfortable with the notion that you have a right to use any medicine that helps your medical condition, regardless of its legal status, you can begin to discreetly explain your situation to friends who might be able to help. It may be embarrassing at first, but consider this. Polling data currently indicates that approximately 70 per cent of Americans approve of patients using marijuana for medical reasons. That figure is even higher in the UK, where one telephone poll showed that 96 per cent of people polled agreed that marijuana should be legalized for medical use. This is a much higher number than most people imagine. So, on average, seven out of ten friends you approach about getting marijuana are likely to already approve of you using it, and that is even before you offer them a detailed explanation.

With many millions of Westerners using marijuana for recreational or medical purposes, there are doubtless hundreds of thousands who are selling it to them. In reality, despite marijuana being illegal, it is fairly common. It is also far safer for you to suffer whatever embarrassment you might feel approaching your friends and acquaintances for help than it is for you to deal with strangers. Networks of marijuana users and suppliers run throughout mainstream society. They are employed in all kinds of occupations, from labourers to professionals. Few think of themselves as criminals. Most of the suppliers typically operate on a small scale and only deal with marijuana. Rather than selling it as their principal livelihood, they are satisfied with modest profits. Some even take satisfaction in simply being a source for their friends. In the same way, many users who purchase only small amounts do occasionally buy a little extra for a friend.

In 1998, a medical marijuana co-operative was set up in Stockport, Greater Manchester. The co-op's founders and associates are part of a growing movement that believes people with recognized medical needs should be able to stock up without resorting to street dealers. The co-op was busted several months later, but the members of the co-op vowed to carry on supplying medicine.

If you are receiving care at a hospital, hospice or other treatment facility, you might have the chance to ask a nurse or other health care worker for help in finding a source for marijuana. Nurses at veterans' hospitals, cancer treatment centres and AIDS treatment centres are often well aware that many of their patients are using marijuana. In some places, health care workers actually wheel their patients outdoors so they can smoke marijuana. It is probably best to only approach a nurse or health care worker with whom you are well acquainted. They might be risking their job to give you the advice you need, and they are likely to be unwilling to take that risk unless they have good reason to trust you.

Fellow patients can also be a source for information about acquiring marijuana. If you participate in a support group for patients with the same or similar medical conditions, you have a good group of prospects to talk to about marijuana. Do not be indiscreet by mentioning it at the first meeting you attend, but do ask other patients how they have dealt with the symptoms you believe might be helped by marijuana. If you are not participating in a patient support group, you might ask your doctor or practice nurse about how to join one.

The very worst way for a patient to get marijuana is to buy it on the street from a stranger. If you are forced to do this, pay attention to a few simple rules. Do not bring a lot of cash or wear expensive jewellery or watches. Purchase small amounts. You will have no way to be certain that what you are buying is actually marijuana, so don't buy a lot of it. Avoid isolated locations where robbery or other violence might take place and go unnoticed. It is probably safer to buy marijuana on a crowded street from someone whispering words like 'buds', 'green', 'smoke', 'leaf', 'pot' or 'hemp' (all slang words for marijuana) as you walk by than it is to make a purchase down a dark deserted alleyway late at night.

Regular users of cannabis are consuming an estimated 800 tonnes of the drug in Britain every year and spending about £3.5 billion on it, according to new research.

A survey of 1,333 regular cannabis users by the independent

drug monitoring unit indicated that regular users spend an average of £68.60 per month on cannabis. Prices are similar throughout the country. The cost of an ounce (25 to 30 grams) of cannabis resin varied between £70 and £120, with an eighth of an ounce of resin costing £15 or less. Skunk, the stronger strain of cannabis, costs between £20 and £25 for the same quantity, home-grown herbal cannabis costs less than half the price of resin.

Another danger patients face in buying marijuana on the street is from police undercover operations in which officers pose as drug sellers. If you are caught in such a way, your penalties are likely to be only for possession. One indication that you may have approached an undercover seller would be if the seller suggests that you buy much more than you asked for or if you are encouraged to do something you had not wanted to do. This might be a sign that you are being enticed to take steps that would expose you to more severe penalties. In fact, most undercover operations are not targeted at buyers but rather at sellers. Officers will pose as buyers seeking out sellers.

Cannabis (Marijuana) Buyers Clubs

The term 'cannabis' is the scientific word for marijuana. Cannabis buyers clubs, or CBCs, are beginning to spring up across the US to meet the needs of patients using marijuana for medical purposes. At present, most CBCs are in California, where the passage of Proposition 215 in 1996 changed state laws to allow patients to use marijuana for medicinal purposes. There are currently about 25 CBCs in California, each serving from 50 to a few thousand patients. Beyond California, we know of CBCs in Washington State, Washington, DC, Oregon, New York and in parts of Canada. No doubt, others exist that we have not yet heard about. There are clubs springing up in the UK, but the police seem to close them down as quickly as they open. Look around, however; regular users will have no doubt located the safest source.

A cannabis buyers club operates somewhat like a pharmacy, except it is technically illegal. However, despite their illegal status, most CBCs operate openly in the US and inform the local authorities of their existence. In many places, police and local officials have become convinced of the sincerity of the people involved and have decided to look the other way, not formally sanctioning the club's activities but not making arrests either. Where clubs have made such arrangements, they have generally instituted strict procedures governing who can obtain marijuana.

In these clubs, patients must provide some evidence, such as a written diagnosis from a doctor, of a medical condition for which marijuana is reasonably believed to be of benefit. The CBC will often try to verify that information by contacting the patient's doctor. The club will also try to determine whether the patient has a doctor's approval for using marijuana. Once patients are approved for membership, they are generally issued some sort of identification card that allows them to gain access to the club later. Marijuana is purchased on the premises. The prices are usually the same as what patients can expect to pay in transactions outside of the club.

In general, CBCs exist where the need is great and where it is possible for providers to step forward and gain the political support needed to continue to operate. While it is necessary for CBCs to have working relationships with the police in their area, they usually also try to build bridges to local health departments and health care providers. The professionalism of many of the CBCs in California cities is widely noted and has led to sufficient political support to permit their continuing operations. Hopefully, this phenomenon will spread to other areas as patients around the world learn more about the potential benefits of marijuana as a medicine. The first UK co-op in Manchester operated on this basis, supplying needy customers with cannabis only after they supplied a doctor's letter confirming diagnosis of a recognized medical condition. Regular clients were given an identification card and signed a document promising not to sell on the drugs.

Marijuana buying clubs or cooperatives also exist underground, as opposed to the CBCs which operate above ground. These underground clubs are usually organized by a single dedicated individual or a small group, who have taken responsibility for supplying medical patients with marijuana at cost. In areas where local officials and police are not cooperative, these underground clubs take precautions to keep their work secret. The best way to find one is through other patients in your area with symptoms or disease syndromes similar to your own.

Chapter 20
What Is the Best Way To Use Marijuana?

Patients who use marijuana for medical purposes must make many decisions for themselves. Since doctors cannot legally prescribe marijuana, the basic choice about whether to use it or not falls to the patient. Since pharmacists cannot sell marijuana, decisions about proper doses and method of administration must also be made by the patient. Finally, since marijuana is an organic plant and not a synthetic chemical, different strains of marijuana may contain variable amounts of active ingredients (cannabinoids) in various combinations. Therefore, patients have to make decisions regarding their source of supply and the degree of consistency they require in the marijuana they need.

If patients are unfamiliar with marijuana, they face a good deal of uncertainty about how to make all of these decisions. This uncertainty can cause stress, discomfort and anxiety. Added to that is the naïve patient's quite understandable fear about acquiring and using an illegal substance like marijuana. Unfortunately, there is no way around this dilemma. That is why so many patients are participating in political efforts to change the laws that prevent them from using marijuana.

Since most surveys have concluded that some 70 million Americans and 6 million people in the UK have smoked marijuana at least once, many readers will not need instruction in how to do it. This chapter is written for the others, and for those with limited experience who may want to consider ways of using marijuana they have not yet tried.

So to begin by answering the question asked in the title of this chapter, there is no best way to use marijuana. If you are going to try it for the first time, or if your experience with it is very limited, you will have to begin by experimenting for yourself. You will need to use trial and error to find the proper dosage, so 'start low and go slow'. You should try different methods of smoking marijuana as well as different ways of putting it in food. We will describe all of your options below. Do not become demoralized or overwhelmed. After some preliminary experimentation, you will find, as most other patients have, that it is relatively easy to gauge the amount of marijuana you will need and the best method for taking it into your body.

The two primary means of delivering marijuana to the body are by smoking or swallowing. Each is physically safe, and each has advantages and disadvantages. For example, smoking marijuana will work best for nausea since it gives immediate relief and allows for accurate dosage control. However, swallowing marijuana may be better for controlling seizures or other symptoms when it is necessary to maintain a constant level of marijuana in one's system in order to ward off the symptoms before they start.

Smoking Marijuana

Smoking is certainly the most common way that patients, as well as recreational users, take marijuana into their bodies. There are a number of ways to smoke marijuana. These include hand-rolled or machine-rolled cigarettes (called 'joints'), standard pipes of various sizes and shapes, with or without filters, and water pipes, some of which are called 'bongs'.

Of the various options for smoking marijuana, the most popular is hand-rolled cigarettes, or joints. Cigarette rolling papers can be bought in almost any shop. Some papers are a little wider than others. They make the joint rolling task a little easier for beginners. You might want to practise first with tobacco. Don't smoke it, just use it to practise rolling cigarettes. You can get rolling tobacco in many shops. Once you have mastered the technique with rolling tobacco, you can move on to rolling joints.

Before rolling the marijuana, you may have to break it down into very small pieces and remove any seeds or sharp pieces of stalk. The seeds will cause uneven burning, acrid smoke and may pop, while the stalks often have sharp edges which may poke through the paper making it difficult to draw smoke. After you prepare a batch of marijuana for rolling, you may want to put two pieces of rolling paper together or use wide rolling papers to give yourself more paper to work with and to make it easier to roll the joint. Do not put as much marijuana into the rolling paper as you would if you were rolling a tobacco cigarette. It is not necessary. Start the joint by curling one edge of the rolling paper over the marijuana. Then roll it forward across the rest of the rolling paper. It will work best if you use two hands and keep your thumbs in the centre of the joint as you roll it. The two outer edges will roll into place if you focus on getting a good roll in the middle of the joint.

Many shops also carry a miniature cigarette rolling device called a 'rolling machine'. This small device will fit into the palm of your hand and cost no more than a few pounds. It consists of a rubber or plastic strip looped over two little cylinders. The width of the rubber strip is about the same as that of the cigarette rolling paper, so the paper fits easily into it. Buy some rolling tobacco and ask the shop assistant to demonstrate the proper technique for using the rolling machine. Once you learn to use it, you can make very neatly rolled joints with no difficulty at all. Some people attempt to put filter tips made from cotton balls into one end of the joint. This is difficult, but you can learn to do it.

Light the joint in the same way you would a cigarette. Drag on it slowly as marijuana does not burn as smoothly as tobacco. If you drag too strongly, the joint is likely to burn unevenly. Because marijuana is so expensive, patients will want to smoke as much of the joint as possible, down to the tiniest stub. Most patients do not throw away any amount of marijuana but rather save the tiny stubs, called 'roaches', and either take them apart so the marijuana that remains can be reused, or stuff them into a pipe and smoke them. Many users have 'roach clips' that they use to hold roaches too small to grasp with the fingers. Tweezers, small pliers, alligator clips or a surgical haemostat will work and allow the user to grasp the small roach and bring it up to the mouth so the joint can be smoked until none of it remains.

Some marijuana users prefer to use a pipe instead of smoking joints. Ordinary tobacco pipes can be used but generally are not preferred because the bowls are too big. Pipes with smaller bowls, specifically designed for marijuana use, can be purchased in many rock music stores or from street vendors if local laws do not allow 'head shops' in your area. These are drug paraphernalia shops, all of which will have a wide variety of marijuana pipes for sale. Home-made filters can be inserted into the stems of any of these pipes to provide a minimal level of protection from a few of the harmful by-products of the smoke.

Smoking marijuana in a pipe is somewhat different from smoking tobacco in a pipe. First, you will need a small screen in the bottom of the pipe. The shards of marijuana will include pieces that are smaller than what is found in pipe tobacco and, as a result, they can be drawn into the pipe stem if there is no screen to prevent that from happening. Purchased marijuana pipes will already have these screens in place. If you need one for a tobacco pipe, you can purchase fine screening materials in a hardware store and cut it to size. The second difference is that it is too wasteful of the marijuana to keep the pipe lit between puffs. It is more economical to relight the pipe with each puff. Because it is illegal, marijuana is very expensive. In fact, with gold currently trading at around $300 (£200) per ounce, marijuana is often worth more than its weight in gold.

A word of caution. Germs can easily collect on pipes, especially on the part you insert into your mouth. Many patients prefer using joints instead of pipes for this reason. As a patient, you may be especially susceptible to infection. If you are going to use a pipe, be sure to thoroughly clean the mouthpiece after each use. You will also have to clean the pipe stem, not so much for germs, but because thick black gunk collects there after prolonged use. It looks like tar and can be removed with ordinary pipe cleaners available wherever cigarettes are sold.

There are several versions of a pocket-sized or collapsible pipe that is often called a 'one-hitter'. It is constructed with a small compartment to store marijuana and a device for smoking it. These one-hitters are very convenient to use and easy to carry around. Their construction prevents most of the smoke that would otherwise escape into the air from doing so. As a result, they can be used discreetly in areas where you might otherwise be reluctant to either openly or even surreptitiously smoke marijuana.

Another way to smoke marijuana is to use a water pipe. This device allows you to draw the smoke through water before inhaling it. Drawing marijuana smoke through water may decrease the amount of impurities inhaled but simultaneously decreases the amount of active ingredients (THC and other cannabinoids) inhaled. Therefore, there may be no net health benefit from using a water pipe except to cool the smoke

(Doblin, 1994). Some people with little or no prior experience smoking tobacco or marijuana find the sometimes difficult task of inhaling smoke a little easier if it is first cooled.

There is a variation of the water pipe, referred to as a 'bong', which allows the user to collect the smoke in a chamber and then inhale it by manipulating an air hole in the pipe. Many recreational marijuana smokers use bongs not simply as water pipes but to collect the smoke from several puffs in the air chamber and then inhale all of it at once. This practice may make it more difficult for patients to regulate their dose, which is one of the most important benefits of smoking marijuana rather than swallowing it.

Swallowing Marijuana

There are many ways of cooking marijuana into food. It can also be made into tinctures and teas, but with greater difficulty. The active ingredients in marijuana are not soluble in water, that is, they do not dissolve in water the way salt or sugar does. Instead they are fat-soluble – they will blend with fat and fatty substances. This is why marijuana persists in the blood for a long time once it is taken into the body (either by smoking or swallowing). Water-soluble substances are more easily flushed out of the body. Because marijuana is fat-soluble, it must be cooked with fats and oils to bring it into solution.

The single most popular way to cook and eat marijuana is by baking it into chocolate brownies. It is also baked into muffins, breads, cookies and cakes, and can be used in various meats and meat loafs, chilli, stuffings, broth, sauces, dips, sweets and ice cream.

There are many books available containing marijuana recipes. We have included some in the list of suggested reading at the back of this book. Excellent recipes can be found in the books by Chris Conrad, Adam Gottlieb, Ed Rosenthal or Tom Flowers that are listed there. You can purchase these and other marijuana cookbooks on the World Wide Web at <http://www.quicktrading.com/>, the site of the Quick Trading Company, which publishes a number of books on marijuana cultivation and cooking. You can also call them at 1-800-428-7825, ext. 102. Recipe books can also be purchased on the web at <http://www.amazon.com/>. Marijuana recipe books are sometimes stocked in bookshops, especially in independently owned bookshops, and are advertised in *High Times* magazine. You can also find many marijuana recipes by searching the web directly using the key words 'marijuana' and 'cook'. Channel Four's *Pot Night* book is available on the web on <http://www.ukcia.org/l.b./research/potnight/>.

One of the principal advantages of cooking with marijuana is that you can carry the food around with you and eat it without revealing that you are using marijuana. Once cooked into a food, it cannot be seen or smelled easily. If you have to use marijuana while at work, or while travelling, or in some other situation where it would be awkward or dangerous to do so, one possible solution is to carry it cooked into a brownie or other food. Some patients also like the fact that when eaten, marijuana is released into the body slowly and over a longer period of time than when it is smoked. This is advantageous for certain conditions, for example epilepsy or spasticity, where marijuana is being used to prevent the onset of symptoms.

The disadvantages of eating marijuana are similar to the disadvantages of swallowing THC (Marinol) or Nabilone pills. It is hard to control dosage, the high is often too powerful, and the effect takes close to an hour to be felt. Other disadvantages are that the cooking can be somewhat complicated and the preparation time can be a minor inconvenience.

When smoking, it is best to use the flowering buds of the marijuana plant because they contain the greatest quantity of THC and other cannabinoids and allow the delivery of more medicine with less smoke. On the other hand, most marijuana cooking is done with the plant's leaves because they tend to be less expensive than buds. Also, the buds contain higher levels of resin and tar which leave a bitter taste in some of the foods that can be prepared with marijuana. Since the leaves contain substantially less THC and other cannabinoids than the buds, you will need a lot of leaves. You will also need to filter out the seeds, stems and stalks before cooking the leaves. All of this adds to the difficulty of cooking marijuana into foods as compared to smoking it in a joint or pipe.

Sterilizing Marijuana

Like any plant material, harvested marijuana will have a certain number of germs, fungi and spores residing upon it. The majority of these organisms are harmless. Those that are not can usually be neutralized by a healthy immune system. Most of these organisms are destroyed when the marijuana is smoked or cooked. Nonetheless, some people believe that there can be exceptions in either instance. There is no scientific evidence to prove this, but since we are discussing marijuana use by patients who may not have healthy immune systems, we want to be extra cautious.

When marijuana burns in a joint or pipe bowl, the heat of the burning material will destroy any organisms living on the material that is being burned. However, some believe that the smoke passing through the remaining marijuana, not yet aflame, may pick up some of the organisms residing there and introduce them into the lungs. There is no proof this can happen, but neither is there proof that it cannot.

When marijuana is cooked in foods, the heat required by the cooking will reliably destroy any bacteria or other organisms present in the marijuana. However, some marijuana recipes call for blending marijuana leaves into food and eating it without cooking. In these cases, any organisms on the marijuana leaves will certainly pass directly into the digestive system and may cause problems. Patients with lowered resistance to infections because of an impaired immune system should avoid eating marijuana in this way.

Since there is a possibility that germs and other organisms can be picked up and transmitted by marijuana smoke, you should seriously consider sterilizing any marijuana before you smoke it, especially if you have an impaired immune system. This can be done with the heat delivered by an oven, a microwave or a tabletop toaster/oven. The main active ingredient in marijuana, THC, begins to break down at about 190°C (374°F). Most dangerous organisms cannot live at temperatures above 71°C (160°F). For example, the pasteurization process used to sterilize milk and other foods takes place at this temperature. Thus, effective sterilization can be achieved by raising the temperature of the marijuana to 71°C (160°F), but no higher than 190°C (374°F).

The best way to achieve this is with an oven or toaster/oven that has an accurate temperature control. The marijuana only needs to be at this temperature for a few minutes. Longer periods are acceptable provided you are sure the temperature control is accurate. Some patients prefer using a microwave because it simultaneously dries the marijuana leaves, making it easier to smoke them. However, temperature control in a microwave is more difficult to achieve. As a result, there is some danger that while effectively sterilizing the marijuana, you will be reducing its potency.

Consult Other Sources about Marijuana

By now, you have learned a great deal about the medicinal properties of marijuana, the advantages and disadvantages of its use and many of the practical considerations you must grapple with should you decide to use it. The final bit of advice we have for you is to continue your education about marijuana. There are hundreds of books and articles about marijuana, with more published each day. Learn as much as you can about the particular aspects of medical marijuana that are important to you.

Many observers believe that patients need to take more responsibility for their own health care. When you use marijuana as a medicine, there is a high probability that you will know more about the medicinal uses of marijuana than your doctor. Its illegal status will force you to get involved and become more knowledgeable than you need to be when you use ordinary prescription medicine. Share your knowledge with your doctor. Suggest books or articles he or she can read to learn more. You will have a much easier time with the difficult decisions you will have to make as the user of an illegal medicine if you can share some of those decisions with your doctor.

In addition, you may want to think about becoming involved in the political battles now taking place to make marijuana available as a legal medicine. You can try to persuade your local elected officials to introduce bills supporting medical marijuana in your borough and city. Write to your local MP, and join one of the growing lobby groups, such as ACT (PO Box CR14, Leeds L57 4XF; Fax 0113 2371000) or the Campaign to Legalize Cannabis International Association (54C Peacock Street, Norwich NR3 1TB; Tel: 01603 625780). However you decide to help in this fight, get involved. It will be good for your health!

References

Baum, D. *Smoke and Mirrors: The War on Drugs and the Politics of Failure.* Boston, Mass: Little, Brown & Co., 1996.

Boulougouris, C. J. et al. 'Social Traits of Heavy Hashish Users and Matched Controls.' *Annals of the New York Academy of Science 282 (1976): 17–23.*

Bowman, M. and R. O. Pihl. 'Cannabis: Psychological Effects of Chronic Heavy Use: A Controlled Study of Intellectual Functioning in Chronic Users of High Potency Cannabis.' *Pharmacologia* 29 (1973): 150–179.

Califano, Joseph A. *The 1996 CASA National Survey of Parents and Teenagers.* New York: Center on Addiction and Substance Abuse, 1996.

Carter, W. E. and P. L. Doughty. 'Social and Cultural Aspects of Cannabis Use in Costa Rica.' *Annals of the New York Academy of Science* 282 (1976): 2–16.

Chang, A. E., D. J. Shiling, R. C. Stillman, et al. 'Delta-9-Tetrahydrocannabinol as an Antiemetic in Cancer Patients Receiving High-Dose Methotrexate.' *Annals of Internal Medicine* 91 (1979): 819–824.

Comitas, L. 'Cannabis and Work in Jamaica: A Refutation of the Amotivational Syndrome.' *Annals of the New York Academy of Science* 282 (1976): 24–32.

Consroe, P. G. Wood and H. Buchsbaum. 'Anticonvulsant nature of marijuana smoking.' *Journal of the American Medical Association* 234 (1975): 306–307.

Dansak, D. A., K. Brazis, E. B. Deaux, et al., Report of the Lynn Pierson Therapeutic Research Program – New Mexico State Department of Health (1986). See <http://www.livelinks.com/nmcu/lptrp.html>

Di Franco, Matthew J. 'The Lack of Association of Marijuana and Other Recreational Drugs with Progression to AIDS in the San Francisco

Men's Health Study.' Paper presented at the XI International Conference on AIDS, Vancouver, BC, Canada, July 1996.

Doblin, R. 'THE MAPS/California NORML Marijuana Waterpipe/ Vaporizer Study.' *Newsletter of the Multidisciplinary Association for Psychedelic Studies* 5 (1994): 1, 19–22.

Doblin, R. and M. Kleiman. 'Marijuana as antiemetic medicine: A survey of oncologists' experiences and attitudes.' *Journal of Clinical Oncology* 9 (1991): 7, 1314–1319.

Dorland's Illustrated Medical Dictionary. 26th edition. Philadelphia, etc. W. B. Saunders, 1981.

Dunn, M. and R. Davis. 'The perceived effects of marijuana on spinal cord injured males.' *Paraplegia* 12 (1974): 175.

Foltin, R. W., J. V. Brady and M. W. Fishman. 'Behavioral analysis of Marijuana effects on food intake in humans.' *Pharmacology, Biochemistry and Behavior* 25 (1986): 577–582.

Formukong, E. A., A. T. Evans and F. J. Evans. 'Analgesic and anti-inflammatory activity of constituents of Cannabis sativa L.' *Inflammation* 12 (1988): 4, 361.

Gowers, W. R. A *Manual of Diseases of the Nervous System*. Vol. 2, 2nd ed. London: J. & A. Churchill, 1893.

Green, L. 'Marijuana effects on intraocular pressure.' *Applied Pharmacology in the Medical Treatment of Glaucomas* (1984) (S.M. Drance, ed.), 507–526.

Grinspoon, L., and J. Bakalar. *Marijuana: The Forbidden Medicine*. New Haven, Conn.: Yale University Press, 1997.

LaGuardia Report. Mayor's Committee on Marijuana. The Marijuana Problem in the City of New York: Sociological, Medical, Psychological and Pharmacological Studies. Lancaster PA: Jacques Cattel Press, 1944.

Mathre, M. L., ed. *Cannabis in Medical Practice: A Legal, Historical and Pharmacological Overview of the Therapeutic Use of Marijuana*. Jefferson, N.C., and London: McFarland & Co., 1997.

Mattison, J. B. 'Cannabis indica as an Anodyne and Hypnotic.' *St Louis Medical Surgical Journal* 61 (1981): 266–267.

McNamara, J. 'The War on Drugs is Lost.' *The National Review*, Feb. 12, 1996. See <http://www.townhall.com/nationalreview/12feb96/contents.html>

Mechoulam, R., ed. *Cannabinoids as Therapeutic Agents*. Boca Raton, Fla.:

CRC Press, Inc., 1986.

Munson, A. E. and K. O. Fehr. 'Immunological Effects of Cannabis,' 257–353 in K. O. Fehr and H. Kalant (eds), *Cannabis and Health Hazards*. Toronto: Addiction Research Foundation, 1983.

Osler, W. *The Principles and Practice of Medicine*, 8th Edition. New York, Appelton, 1913.

Page, J. B., et al. 'Psychosociocultural Perspectives on Chronic Cannabis Use: The Costa Rican Follow-up,' *Journal of Psychoactive Drugs* 20 (1988): 57–65.

Petro, D. and C. Ellenberger, Jr. 'Treatment of human spasticity with delta-9-tetrahydrocannabinol.' *Journal of Clinical Pharmacology* 21 (1981): 413S–416S.

Randall, R. C., ed. *Cancer Treatment and Marijuana Therapy*. Washington, DC: Galen Press, 1990.

Rosenbaum, M., *Kids, Drugs, and Drug Education: A Harm Reduction Approach*. National Council on Crime and Delinquency, 1996.

Rosenthal, E., D. Gieringer and T. Mikuriya. *Marijuana Medical Handbook: A Guide to Therapeutic Use*. Oakland, California: Quick American Archives, 1997.

Salan, S. E., N. E. Zinberg and E. Frei. 'Anti-emetic effect of delta-9-tetrahydrocannabinol in patients receiving cancer chemotherapy.' *New England Journal of Medicine* 293 (1975): 16, 795–797.

Silverstein, M. J. and P. Lensin. '2, 4-Dinitrochlorobenzene Skin Testing in Chronic Marijuana Users,' 199–203, in M. C. Braude and S. Szara (eds), *Pharmacology of Marijuana*. New York: Raven Press, 1976.

Vinciguerra, V., T. Moore and E. Brennan. 'Inhalation marijuana as an antiemetic for cancer chemotherapy.' *NY State Journal of Medicine* 88 (1988): 525–527.

Zimmer, L. and J. P. Morgan. *Marijuana Myth, Marijuana Facts: A Review of the Scientific Evidence*. New York: The Lindesmith Center, 1997.

Suggested Reading

Books

The Art and Science of Cooking With Cannabis: The Most Effective Methods of Preparing Food & Drink With Marijuana, Hashish & Hash Oil by Adam Gottlieb (Ronin Publishing, 1993).

Cancer Treatment & Marijuana Therapy edited by R. C. Randall (Galen Press, 1990).

Cannabinoids as Therapeutic Agents edited by Raphael Mechoulam, PhD (CRC Press, Inc. 1986).

Cannabis in Medical Practice: A Legal, Historical, and Pharmacological Overview of the Therapeutic Use of Marijuana edited by Mary Lynn Mathre, RN (McFarland & Company, Inc. 1997)

From Chocolate to Morphine: Everything You Need to Know about Mind-Altering Drugs by Andrew Weil, MD, and Jennifer Rosen (Houghton Mifflin, 1983 and 1993).

Grandpa's Marijuana Handbook: A User guide for Ages 50 & Up by Evan Keliher (Pedagogue Press, 1997).

The Great Book of Hemp by Rowan Robinson (Park Street Press, 1996).

Hemp for Health: The Medicinal and Nutritional Uses of Cannabis Sativa by Chris Conrad (Healing Arts Press, 1997).

HEMP: *Lifeline to the Future* by Chris Conrad (Chris Conrad, 1994).

Marijuana: The Forbidden Medicine by Lester Grinspoon, MD, and James Bakalar, JD (Yale University Press, 1997).

Marijuana Reconsidered by Lester Grinspoon, MD (Harvard University Press, 1971 and 1977 and Lester Grinspoon 1994 and Quick American Archives, 1996)

Marijuana and AIDS: Pot, Politics & PWAs in America by R.C. Randall (Galen Press, 1991).

Marijuana Botany by Robert Connell Clarke (Ronin Publishing, 1992).

Marijuana Grower's Guide by Mel Frank (Red Eye Press, 1997).

Marijuana Grower's Handbook by Ed Rosenthal (Bookpeople, 1991).

Marijuana Grower's Insider's Guide by Mel Frank (Red Eye Press, 1989).

Marijuana Herbal Cookbook by Tom Flowers (Quick Trading Publication, 1996).

Marijuana Medical Handbook: A Guide to Therapeutic Use by Ed Rosenthal, Dale Gieringer, PhD, and Tod Mikuriya, MD (Quick American Archives, 1997).

Marijuana: Medical Papers 1839–1972 edited by Tod H. Mikuriya, MD (Medi-Comp Press, 1973).

Marijuana Myths, Marijuana Facts: A Review of the Scientific Evidence by Lynn Zimmer, PhD, and John Morgan, MD (The Lindesmith Center, 1997)

Muscle Spasm, Pain & Marijuana Therapy edited by R. C. Randall (Galen Press, 1991).

National Drug Strategy: The Health and Psychological Consequences of Cannabis Use, Monograph 25 of The Drug Offensive (Australian Government Printing Services, 1995).

Smoke and Mirrors: The War on Drugs and the Politics of Failure by Dan Baum (Little, Brown, 1996).

Medical Journal Articles

American Public Health Association Endorsement on Medical Marijuana (*American Journal of Public Health*, March 1996, vol. 86, no. 3, pp. 441–442). See <http://www.natlnorml.org/medical/alpha.endorse.html>

'Deglamorising Cannabis' (editorial in *The Lancet*, vol. no. 346, no. 8985, 11 Nov. 1995). See <http://www.xs4all.nl/~mlap/press/lancet1.html>

'Federal Foolishness and Marijuana' by Jerome Kassirer, MD (*New England Journal of Medicine*, vol. 336, no. 16, 30 Jan. 1997, pp. 366–367). See<http://www.nejm.org/public/1997/0336/0005/0366/1. htm>

'Marihuana as Medicine: A Plea for Reconsideration' by Lester Grinspoon, MD, and James Bakalar, JD. (*Journal of the American Medical Association*, vol. 273, no. 23, 21 June 1995, pp. 1875–1876). See <http://www.pdxnorml.org/JAMA_M_as_Medicine_062195.html>

'Marijuana as Antiemetic Medicine: A Survey of Oncologists' Experience and Attitudes' by Richard Doblin and Mark Kleiman (*Journal of Clinical Oncology*, vol. 9, no. 7, July 1991, pp. 1314–1319). See

<http://www.pdxnorml.org/JOCO_antiemetic_070191.html>

'Reefer Madness – The Federal Response to California's Medical-Marijuana Law' by George Annas, JD MPH (*New England Journal of Medicine*, vol. 337, no. 6, 7 Aug. 1997, pp. 435–439). See <http://www.nejm.org/public/1997/0337/0006/0435/1.htm>

'The War on Drugs' (editorial in the *British Medical Journal*, vol. 311, Dec. 1995, pp. 23–30. See <http://www.xs4all.nl/~mlap/press/bmj1.html>

Websites

Alliance for Cannabis Therapeutics <http://www.marijuana-as-medicine.org/>

Campaign to Legalize Cannabis International Association <http://www.uk/cia/groups/clcia/clcia.html/>

The Drug Policy Foundation <http://www.dpf.org/>

Drug Reform Coordination Network <http://www.drcnet.org/>

Drug Reform Coordination Network Online Library of Drug Policy <http://www.druglibrary.org>

International Coalition to Legalize Cannabis <http://www.schmoo.co.uk/mayday.html>

International Cannabinoid Research Society <http://www.129.49.19.42/ICRS/ICRS_main.html>

The Lindesmith Center <http://www.lindesmith.org/>

Marijuana and the War on (some) Drugs <http://www.calyx.net/marijuana.html>

Multidisciplinary Association for Psychedelic Studies, Inc. <http://www.maps.org/>

National NORML Homepage <http://www.natlnorml.org/>

New Mexicans for Compassionate Use <http://www.livelinks.com/nmcu>

Portland NORML Homepage <http://www.pdxnorml.org/>

UKCIA (UK Cannabis Information) <http://www.ukcia.org/>

Who Supports Access to Medical Marijuana? <http://www.marijuana-as-medicine.org/support.html>

Books not available in your local bookshop may be ordered through http://www.amazon.com.

Index

Bold type indicates main or substantial entries